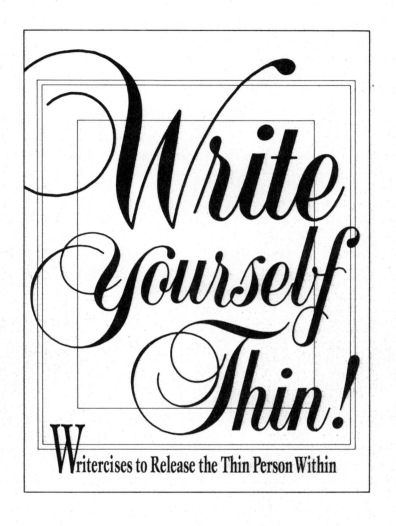

Write Yourself Thin!

Writercises to Release the Thin Person Within

Toni Lynn Allawatt

CompCare® Publishers

2415 Annapolis Lane
Minneapolis, MN 55441

Library of Congress Cataloging-in-Publication Data
Allawatt, Toni Lynn, 1950-
    Write Yourself Thin by Toni Lynn Allawatt.
      p. cm.
    ISBN 0-89638-238-9
    1. Reducing—Psychological aspects.
  2. Writing—Psychological aspects. I. Title.
RM222.2.A393 1990
616.85'2606—dc20   90-22020
                                                                CIP

Cover and interior design by Susan Rinek

Inquiries, orders, and catalog requests should be addressed to
CompCare Publishers
2415 Annapolis Lane
Minneapolis, Minnesota 55441
Call toll free 1-800-328-3330
(Minnesota residents call 1-612-559-4800)

6	5	4	3	2	1
96	95	94	93	92	91

For my mother and father, who loved me through thick and thin, and for my daughter Jess, who brought out the skinny kid in me. For Nancy Kovats Lea, who encouraged me to write and teach; for Christine Staruch Ferguson, who inspired me to dream, dream, dream; and for Steven "Ingo" Milton, who cared about my fat feelings.

Contents

Introduction

I kept my first diary at the age of six. It was one of those types with a lock and the days marked off. I had made much preliterate scribbling amid one solitary entry.

In chicken-scrawl letters I wrote, "I like Toni."

Maybe if I'd have penned that every day for the next thirty years, I wouldn't have grown discontented and overweight.

Later journals, it turned out, were filled with self-deprecating junk. As the food of the same persuasion fills me with empty calories, so writing from the bottomless pit of self-pity leaves me full of anger and resentment.

At thirty-six years old and pushing 175 pounds, I felt inked out and out of control. Also, I felt desperate. I'd recently had an artificial knee replacement, which meant that my extra baggage was weighing heavily upon my new joint, causing much swelling and discomfort.

I wanted to *be* different, *feel* different, but I didn't know how to change. I was carrying around more than extra pounds. I was loaded down with emotional flab and knew that even six months on the "Rice Diet" wouldn't remove cellulite of the psyche.

Too bad I couldn't afford expensive therapy.

However, since writing had always been therapeutic for me, it seemed logical to enlist my creativity to reshape the way I viewed my body and, at the very least, accept myself in my overweight condition. And then there was always the hope that maybe, just maybe, the daily exercise of diary writing would help me rewrite the emotional score, balance the scale, flesh out my Thin Woman, and get my Fat Lady in control.

Anaïs Nin, the famous French diarist, said, "Neurosis is nothing more than blocked creativity." Since I had a neurotic attitude about food, perhaps my creativity would accomplish what years of willpower could not.

On November 5, 1986, I wrote on the cover of a spiral notebook "Diary of a Fat Lady." It sounded ironic and funny. I liked it because I knew that in order to succeed, I would have to call off the war, befriend my Fat Lady, serenade my Thin Woman.

"Come out, come out, wherever you are," I wrote on that first empty page.

Two notebooks later, I trimmed down to 129 muscular pounds. The journal writing worked better than a trip to a fat farm.

I am now in the body I want to be in. There seems little likelihood of gaining the weight back, unless I write the exercises in reverse.

Diary writing worked because, more than the physical scars I carried from the old motorcycle accident that injured my knee, emotional wounds were keeping me fat. The diary was a safe way to pick at the scabs of my feelings without the threat of digging too deep and drawing blood. Discovery, however, is only half the story. The real magic in writing my "Diary of a Fat Lady" lay in plotting a happier, healthier ending.

Almost any diet will work to take weight off. But the secret to get and stay thin is to feel and think thin.

I did and you can too.

You can condition yourself to turn to your diary instead of a snack. Writing can spell out your hunger for what it often is—an inner desire for emotional fulfillment rather than physical sustenance. Fashioning a new body takes more than willpower and self-sacrifice—it takes a little imagination. Writing about fat fears and skinny scenarios is not only creative, but fun and habit-forming.

Even though my weight has stabilized for the last several years, I continue to write letters of love and hope to both my Fat

Lady and Thin Woman. I believe that the more understanding you accord that part of yourself I call your Fat Lady, the healthier and happier you can become.

When my weight dropped noticeably, friends and acquaintances began asking how I did it. I explained about my diaries. A very dear friend encouraged me to organize my diaries into systematic exercises. That was the beginning of my showing many others how to chart their own maps to Slimtown.

Looking over my diaries I found them full of self-help techniques—positive thinking, visual imagery, relaxation fantasies, neurolinguistic programming, and affirmations. In 1988, I opened my home to women who wanted to get in touch with their Fat Ladies and Thin Women. From those parlor sessions evolved my Thinkercise workshops, which use creative visualization and writing exercises, "writercises," to shape a better body image and imagine a better body shape.

This book is organized into two parts. Part 1 chronicles my personal heavyweight history and liberation to life as a lightweight. While Part 1 is my own private soap opera, Part 2 is detailed script from my Thinkercise workshops. This is where you'll find writercises that will teach you to write yourself thin. If you are motivated and ready to write, by all means skip the drama and dig right into writercising.

If, however, writing yourself thin sounds to you like growing slim by studying chemistry or subtracting weight the algebra way, you might want to do as the comedian Sid Caesar did.

After his initial rise to fame and fortune, he crashed through the roof of depression and alcoholism. When traditional therapy failed to uncover the root of his unhappiness, Sid Caesar turned to a tape recorder to play the silent role of therapist.

What he uncovered was bizarre.

He remembered being an infant, rolling uncontrollably down, down, down—until, like magic, something reached out and stopped the roller coaster. While he couldn't figure the source, he connected these free-falling experiences to the panic that his high-flying success engendered. All during his famous years, he kept expecting a fist to reach out and knock him off the mountain.

Upon further digging, an older brother admitted to tying a rope to baby Sid's stroller and letting it hurl full-speed down a long, steep hill. The mysterious hand that had made Sid so insecure was his brother, reeling the stroller back.

Shortly after this discovery, Sid Caesar got his life together and staged a comeback.

If writing has little appeal to you, I would suggest that you do the writercises with a tape recorder. Talk yourself into— and through—this marvelous journey of self-discovery. Either way, thinkercising or writercising can help you to change the way you perceive yourself. And thinking thin is the first step toward being thin.

I once heard an editor of *Big Beautiful Woman* magazine say that most women who lose weight gain it back quickly because they still own that weight. Your diary is a way to disown your weight while still claiming the Fat Lady beneath your surface. Tracking your Fat Lady can ultimately lead you to your Thin Woman.

I realize that the word *fat* may sound derogatory to some. However, I found that using the word frequently, especially when I was at my fattest, made it a friendlier term. Why shouldn't we call ourselves fat? Why not take the word back from those who use it derisively and give it respect?

Finding dignity in my fat encouraged a truce between my Fat Lady and Thin Woman.

And now, please indulge me as I make this entry in your book to tell my own story. Hopefully, something you read here will inspire you to begin writing your own weight-loss story, and yours will be able to end with a similar sign-off:

I like Toni

Part 1

Diary of a Fat Lady

Ode to My Fat Lady

*Your overstated hips speak to me
in melodramatic sign language
bulging with possibilities . . .*

November 5, 1986

1

Getting to Know Me

Chubby in Pink

I wasn't always fat.

As a matter of fact I was a thin teen-ager.

But there was this skirt—a pleated, pink linen—that I wore through the eighth grade. It made me *feel* chubby. That was back in the early sixties when the fashion industry was just beginning its cold war on size twelve and I was just entering the palestra of puberty. Every time I put on that skirt, I felt like a blimp.

Recording this, my primal fear of fat, I wrote:

November 20, 1986

My hips aren't any bigger underneath these pink pleats. How come I feel like the circus fat lady? How come I feel trapped inside the incredible ballooning pleats? Why does it seem fat will eventually sabotage all my pursuit?

I remember how a family friend once joked about women who were overweight.

"Don't ever get fat," she said. "People will stare at you in restaurants to see how much you eat. Boys will want you to ask the girl of their dreams out for them, and when you get older, other women will expect you to babysit their children because you have nothing better to do."

To me, fat had always meant eating alone, living alone and loving alone.

Now if I close my eyes and put on that pink skirt, I feel my skinny thirteen-year-old hips pushing out those pleats. I feel my Chubby Child pleading, "Never, ever get fat."

"I feel hungry, so hungry, yet I better not eat. Other people will count the bites." That's what I thought then. So instead I would sneak potato chips on the long walk home from school.

I felt like I could only eat alone.

Maybe it was that pink skirt that made me hate my Catholic high school's pleated plaid uniform. Four years of wearing pleats day after day, feeling like a solemn, holy hog. I bet I only weighed 110 pounds, yet I felt fat all the time. And then sitting in the gym, eating my lunch on my lap because the school had no cafeteria, I would try to hide my package of cookies inside a pleat so no one would know I was indulging my sweet tooth.

I was thin then. Too bad I never really enjoyed it. Next time I'm thin I'm going to enjoy every step I take, every morsel I eat.

And next time I'm feeling fat, I'm going to invite a few friends over for food-for-all. I'm going to put on a pink skirt and insist they watch me eat. I'm going to stare at myself in the mirror and tell myself I feel healthy in pink, I look pretty in pleats.

I didn't actually pig out in front of the world. Instead I focused on relaxing myself whenever I ate in public. I would take a deep breath and tell myself, "I look healthy in pink pleats. I look lovely with food filling my cheeks."

Acting out a fear is the quickest way I know to show it for what it is—a heavy emotional burden. And dead weight is about as useful as hot ice.

Scarred and Scared

Eventually, however, I really did get fat.

And more than once.

The first time my Fat Lady took over I was twenty-one. A motorcycle accident had left me in a body cast for six months and hip-length casts for another year and a half. Inactivity made the takeover inevitable. My Fat Lady easily usurped my Thin Woman's tenuous hold.

When I was off crutches, a well-meaning family doctor gave me diet pills to help me lose the excess pounds gained while my leg was broken, yet no one knew what to give me to mend my broken spirit.

There is something about a traumatic injury that confirms the darkest of self-doubts and deepest of self-recriminations.

November 25, 1986

When they cut that final cast off, I looked at this shriveled, hairy, crusty, brown leg, dented with scars and shaped like a twisted tree limb, and I remember crying later into my pillow. I felt I had to pretend it didn't matter. I'd already put my parents through enough anguish. I had to be strong, make like I didn't care—after all, I was the smart sister. What did a gimp leg matter to a bookworm? I'd never planned on a beauty queen career anyway.

Oh, but the horror of wearing a bathing suit! I remember going to the beach that first time with Maureen. She looked like a *Seventeen* magazine model and I limped along, plump and peculiar. I felt every eye staring at my leg as if it were neon orange.

And the saddest part of all was that even before the accident which gnarled my knee, I'd hated my fat knees . . .

Diary entries such as this focused the feelings of alienation and eccentricity I had from the injury. Yet, the more I probed, the more I realized my leg only highlighted a deeper inferiority. For some reason I'd always suspected I wasn't worthy of joy. I didn't deserve to be thin.

The summer of my eleventh year I spent searching the fields near my home, looking for mutant four leaf clovers. I think that I believed I was going to need a whole lot of luck to make it through life. The many four- and few five-leaf clovers I did find, I pressed into an old copy of *The Hunchback of Notre Dame*.

After the accident I identified more with Quasimodo than with the beautiful prisoner. Early in the diary I wrote the following letter to my Fat Lady:

December 3, 1986

Dear Fat Lady,

Who are you?
You are soft as a bed pillow. Do you cushion my falls? Are you afraid of falling? Failing? Do you protect me from rejection? No one will notice the scars through all this fat.
How truly kind of you.
But you don't need to hide me from the world anymore. I am ready to be exposed. I want to give my knee the healthiest, thinnest body possible. I know I can follow a diet and exercise program—up to a point. I need your help to get me past my turn-off point.
Think about this, my Fat Lady friend: In story writing, I often reach a similar crisis, times when I doubt my own talent.
"I'm a crummy writer. Why bother?"
Yet, instead of flicking on the television and switching off the computer, instead of crying, "What's the difference—I'm no Virginia Woolf," instead, I write through the despair. I keep on producing more

crummy prose until I come around to believing in my verse again.

Fat Lady/Thin Woman, do you feel that you are always going to have gnarled scars so why bother getting thin? If thin is beautiful and scars are ugly, then perhaps you believe I can never be thin and beautiful, and so you save me from disappointment.

Yet I say that scars are beautiful.

Scars are merely a road map of where I've been.

Scars are yesterday's teardrops.

My scars are my link to the sky. I had to skid across the ground in order to look up and kiss the clouds and open my mind once more to God. How could all that be ugly?

Fat Lady, I thank you for protecting me, but I no longer need the insulation of fat.

Let my fat burn into energy.

Thank you.

Ever Yours,

I mailed that letter to myself and read it often. The more I read it, the more comfortable I became with my scars. I continued writing to my scars, trying to set right the twisted perspective branded upon my spirit by my imperfect flesh. Slowly, I kneaded the cicatrix and loosened the scar tissue's hold upon my emotions.

That's the miracle of journal writing. It heals by laying open the real problem like a wound needing air. Sometimes you have to read between the lines, but it's all there.

Much later I wrote letters to my scars, thanking them for closing the wounds, serenading them with poetry. After all, my scars will be with me a lifetime and I want to love every part of myself. (Although I have had one scar reconstructed through plastic surgery, the others do not lend themselves to skin grafts.)

Releasing my feelings about flesh and bone wounds left me free to address other kinds of scars, the invisible yet truly debilitating ones: my disfigured feelings about myself.

Slow, Stop, Yield

Skid-marked skin, you speak to me of
potholes and cracked curbs
and detours in the dark,
fate-mined tolls,
and twisted lanes,
and bridges blown apart.
Vulnerable skin
opening
to the cold chrome
and hot tar,
disjointed voices
raining like static from
a schizophrenic radio dial,
a friend crying
"are-re-re
you-ou-ou
hur-ur-urt?"

Later, all those gangrene masks
watching, waiting,
poking, probing
I heard my father give
permission to amputate
and I willed those wounds to weld together
to scar me back
into a waking whole.
O, graceful cicatrix,
why do I curse you
when you were born to save me
the anguish of walking
on wood.

Action Speaks Louder Than Words

As a writer I knew that in fiction, the events of plot must lead to revelation, and revelation to change. My diary writing was certainly revealing much about my fat fears and thin hopes, but what about change?

It is action that makes the final statement, twists the events into a surprise, or turns a life around.

I needed to do more than just write inner dialogues. I needed to plot believable solutions to my problems and then, like any good character, stick to my own script.

On December 5, I started eating more nitty-gritty meals, consisting of whole grains, fruits, vegetables, and low-fat protein. I also joined a health club.

Ever since my knee-replacement surgery, I'd been exercising at home, using various workout videos and a stationary bike; however, the glaring mirrors of a health club reflected so many fit and trim bodies, I experienced a relapse:

December 10, 1986

Why am I afraid to exercise in front of the class? I prefer watching the instructor close up. My reflection in that front mirror inspires me to kick higher. Watching myself keeps me better balanced.

And yet I feel I don't belong up front, as if that first row was a throne to be won by a shapely body and perfect balance. Maybe mirrors belong to youth and beauty.

Up front, everyone can see my clumsiness. Up front I can see my awkward struggles with fitness and fat. Maybe people behind me would rather look at a better body.

So what! So what that I'm clumsy and awkward and a bit of a gimp. Maybe my struggles will encourage someone with a bad back or too much fat to move closer to the mirrors. So let it be.

Perhaps the younger girls, the perfect bodies, do consider me the fat lady who blocks their view of themselves. But as long as there is an empty spot up front, I've already paid my dues to be there. The front lines will always evoke controversy.

Be brave and dare the mirrors.

For, in truth, the more I work out in front of the mirrors, the less grotesque my reflection seems.

Don't Be So Quick to Bake Me

So what I'm fat!
I do not live on additives
nor artificial hearts
and candy-coated lies
So what I'm big and round!
I do not gorge on the rib-eye
nor the cold cut
of someone else's pie.
I'm not lean and I'm not mean!
nor am I a jolly jelly roll
sweeter than a dumpling yam
in a marshmallow bowl.
So what I'm fat!
look beyond my dough
and past your doubt
to the surprise inside.

Mirror, Mirror in My Diary

The drama that played within my diary challenged my Fat Lady to change. Every day I felt less and less like the villain of my own body. In the beginning I wrote often, sometimes two or three times a day. I kept my diary in a drawer in the kitchen, so it could be a convenient detour whenever I strolled into the danger zone.

17

December 4, 1987

I want more of those chocolate chip oatmeal cookies I baked. Two is not enough. I'm angry at you, Fat Lady. If I hadn't stopped here to write, you'd have bargained me into another, and another. You convinced me that one little taste would be enough—but it never is enough, is it?

You fat pig!

There I said it. And now that it's out on paper, I see how intolerant I am. I have more tolerance than to curse my appetite.

I'm munching out of boredom. There's a world of things to do besides eat. I can take a bike ride to the park. Yes. And I'm sorry I called myself a fat pig. I am a Thin Woman with self-control and self-esteem.

Often the last thing I felt like doing was writing in that notebook. Still I kept opening the drawer instead of the refrigerator. I told myself that, if after a page of writing I continued to need a snack, I could have something.

Sometimes writing wasn't enough. And sometimes I ignored the drawer and went straight for the food pump.

"Fill 'er up," the Fat Lady would order.

After another similar slip, I wrote an angry epistle to the "fat fanatic who sabotaged my rescue mission." After the rage, I asked her why. This was her only reply:

"Because I am not perfect."

I apologized and never wrote her off like that again. Slowly, my big binges became little larks as my hand jogged along the lines of notebook paper, exercising tired memories.

Mostly I wrote to the Fat Lady, asking her if she was really physically hungry. Sometimes I'd write persuasive essays on why she only thought she was hungry.

December 9, 1987

C'mon, Fat Lady, you're not really hungry. You go to the fridge pretending to be just browsing. Two or three times you come and peak inside, still feigning casual interest. Then, WHAM, you grab the ice cream.

But the truth is, you're not physically hungry. All those healthy meals fill up you up quite nicely.

You've just got the eating habit. Food is your diversion from momentary boredom. Food keeps your mouth busy. Maybe you're afraid you might tell someone why you're rolling in fat. That you're hoping men won't spot you behind the eight ball. If one did, you might take a shot and scratch.

Just now, watching "Moonlighting," you had a stray thought about walking on the beach with that last boyfriend before the crash. It was easy then to wear a bathing suit. Now it's harder than squeezing into a size eight bikini.

Does your past love life make you sad? Send you searching through the cookie jar? Don't worry, there'll be more walks on the beach again, sometime, somewhere.

Besides, food only makes life feel better for the time it takes to chew it. The wrong food or even too much of the right stuff leaves behind a bad taste in your mind. A dull ache.

When you were younger, you hated all things dull—dull conversations, colors, books, clothes, dreams—and especially dull people. Think about how much food dulls you. Instead of stimulating your brain, your blood is busy digesting all those heavy calories.

C'mon, Fat Lady, let's give the Thin Woman another chance, one more stroll on the beach, another glimpse through the rose-colored sunglasses.

Although that particular entry touched the tip of my sexual iceberg, I wasn't yet ready to go exploring my frozen tundra. I knew I had serious problems with men that kept my Thin Woman hidden within. Being a single mother, I knew firsthand about laboring over the pain of separation. Yet, it would be many, many months before I was ready to thaw out my hardened heart.

Nothin' Says Lovin' Like Somethin' from Mom's Oven

Those first few months of journaling, I really got to know every dimple in the cellulite, to understand every growl of my Fat Lady's stomach. I learned that hunger isn't always satisfied by something as simple as buttered toast.

At one point, my Fat Lady admitted to seeking success in the sweet concoctions she sometimes smuggled into the house. Cream puffs reminded her of the lemon pudding cupcakes my mother made to help me forget every minor disappointment of my young life and chocolate reminded me of Mom's fudge.

Like exploring a cavity with a curious tongue, my pen probed the emotional chemistry of my sweet tooth. Often my desire for sugar dissolved by pouring ink on the real longing. Also, writing childish references to "Mommie" seemed to be a more direct line to the innocence of truth.

December 10, 1986

Dear Fat Lady,

I'm tired of working on a novel that probably will never be published. I'm tired of putting words together in order to prove my worth. I would rather run home to Mommie and have her bake me up a batch of cupcakes.

Mommie loves me no matter how many books I write.

When I was little, just knowing there was some goodie in the oven was enough to comfort me. Beside the sweet tastes, I wonder about the meaning of Mommie baking. Maybe I simply long to climb back into her oven, let her bake me again for nine long months.

Never have to think then.

Ah, but I love to think. I love to write and think—and yet, right now I would love to climb into a nice warm oven and neither write nor think. But not necessarily for nine months.

Ah, that's it. The truth is, I'm more tired than hungry.

I miss Mom. I'll always miss Mom, but eating's not going to move her any closer. Instead of staying up any later, writing and thinking about cupcakes and cream puffs, I'm going to curl into an embryonic cuddle and sleep, sleep, sleep.

Maybe I can dream a dream of Mommie.

And so I did. As I turned more and more to my diary for comfort and less and less to food, I began to realize that although I lived half a country away from my relatives, my eating was still very much a family affair.

Guess Who's Coming to the Dinner Table?

During the two years that I was actively editing my body, I wrote extensively about my primary family dinner table, including my sisters, Cathy, Patty, and Fran, recalling who sat where and who said what.

June 3, 1987

I sat across from Cathy. Her healthy appetite contrasted with my own fussy eating habits. I was a real peanut butter kid and bologna sandwich binger. How frustrated my mother would get when I scraped the sauce and cheese from pizza and picked the peppers from my meat loaf. I guess my finicky eating got me the attention I needed.

I wish to let go of all those controlling habits attached to food.

I wish to think of food for its nutrient value . . .

I continued exploring that family dinner table, especially those special occasions, those holiday meals loaded with fattening foods and sometimes, explosive emotions.

A few months after beginning my journal journey into my Fat Lady's consciousness, I returned to my family home for a Christmas visit.

I felt nervous about returning to old tempers and temptations, yet armed with my diary, I planned to observe and record the family dynamics that originally molded my eating patterns. Enlightenment, I hoped, of both pounds and insights was just an airplane ride away.

The following is but one of many revelations I brought back with me from my family dinner table. I wasn't actually sitting there scribbling in my diary from under the table as this may sound—I wrote this after the meal. However, I prefer to write in the present tense whenever possible. It helps me be more in the moment.

Also, psychologists agree that the subconscious mind listens for cues about the present. In other words, if you use the future tense, telling yourself that "I will be thinner tomorrow," your subconscious and your body understand this direction as "sometime in the future I want to change but for now—do nothing."

For in the subconscious mind, tomorrow never comes.

December 25, 1986

For the first time I feel a new kind of dinner table "etiquette"—I feel my emotions in control. There is something calming and powerful watching me be myself. I feel a sense of choice. I don't need to behave in my old, set ways.

I watch as my parents play their roles. My mother dances around the table, waiting on everyone. I wonder how her servility affects my own eating patterns. I guess I feel guilty, so I keep eating to show my participation in the family. For at least a decade now we sisters have urged her to sit with us, yet how many meals before that did I place my orders for milk and mayonnaise, knives and napkins? I carry this guilt like a stolen tip and yet, I see now that Mother chooses her own position. Though I wish she would join us, I am not responsible for her choice.

I here and now let go of my guilt.

There, that helps.

I continue to watch as Daddy jokes and teases one or the other of his four daughters. The only man at the table, he is like the centerpiece. We four sisters vie for his attention. I grow shyer with every meal.

The oldest and the youngest steer the conversation. My other middle sister and I occasionally add a bit of wit. She is much better at that than I am. She makes everyone laugh. I want to shovel in more food—to stuff down my sensitivity to keep from feeling left out, to have something to do rather than merely stare at the animation around me.

This time, however, I do not.

This time I have a choice. This time I allow myself to watch and smile. This time I tell myself that, of course, I am a vital part of this family scene. My quietness is as much my choice as are my occasional comments. It is okay to watch and observe. It was my reflective temperament that molded me into a writer. I am grateful to the part my family dynamics had in giving me this.

I hereby let go of any resentment I might hold
toward Daddy for wielding the power to notice or not
to notice me. I herewith let go of the jealousy I feel
for my sisters, for their wit or my lack of it.

I let go of my self-denigration for my
dinner-table demureness.

In the years since then I have felt much more relaxed
during holiday visits. Although I continue to bring my diary, I
only need to write a few analytical or affirming lines, sometimes
before and sometimes after dinner.

It helps keep me honest.

Putting a New Picture of Me in the Family Album

After crutches and college I moved West, far away from family
dinners and Mom's cupcakes. Yet, no matter how far I wandered,
my first family was never far from my inner table.

I came from a nice, if a bit overly protective family, yet
even the most "normal" of families leave uncomfortable brands
upon the heart—and stomach.

The diary left me free to rant and rail against real and
imagined injustices. Knowing no one would ever see it, it left
me free to howl and bitch like a witch of a she-wolf. This kind
of cathartic writing rid me of much bitterness and anger that
would have otherwise poisoned my appetite for life. I did try,
however, never to close my notebook on a downbeat, but rather
to keep writing until I could see the other side of the picture.

While in the throes of a midnight nibble-a-thon, I mumbled about my siblings and wrote out my middle-child melancholia.

February 18, 1987

. . . Sitting at the kitchen table is the comfort here.
The comfort is in the big round table, the bright
overhead light.
　　Why?
　　I remember all those boring Sunday afternoons
sitting around the table with my sisters, drawing
pictures and escaping into the construction paper of
pastel fans or the newsprint of paper maché masks,
coloring Easter eggs, or drawing rows of Betty Boops
wearing the latest fashions.
　　My sisters seem to have made their lives
continuing works-in-progress. My life feels like the
third draft of an unfinished novel. Of course, Patty
would tell me we are all the same.
　　That's what I'm craving. Not hunks of cheese
globbed with peanut butter. I miss the colors, the
textures, the act of making my fantasies visual. I miss
my sisters.
　　There. Now I can sit in the kitchen and feed
the real hunger. Now I can draw a portrait of my Thin
Woman. Now I control my own outline. I can trace
my shape, fat or thin. The design is mine. I can send a
picture of my Fat Lady off to my sisters and we can
laugh and cry about all the fat ladies who float in and
out of our dreams.

The more I isolated the real hungers, the more the imagined ones lost their bite.

I did draw a picture of myself. First, I drew my Fat Lady and put a smile on her. I told her it was time to thin down and hoped she understood. Then with a pair of scissors I pared my paper doll of her excesses.

Thin Linnie in Blue Jeans

I colored that paper doll yellow and blue and slipped her into the pocket of a pair of jeans I hadn't worn since 1983. Soon after that, I began writing to the Thin Woman who seemed to live inside of me. I believe that just as there was a young Fat Lady in my thin pink pleats, so there was a Thin Woman inside this fat body waiting for me to invite her to her own coming-out party.

In the beginning the Fat Lady had so much to say, she dominated my diary. I could feel her, heavy and solid, inside me. The character of my Thin Woman seemed wispier, harder to imagine. When I wrote from her perspective, I felt like I was faking her. Yet I found the more I pretended, the more real she felt, and the more I adopted the lifestyle that nurtured thinness.

So what if I was only a Fat Lady pretending to be a thin one. My steps grew lighter and slowly my body began to conform. I shed 10 pounds just playing at being thin.

Five months after I began tracking my fat feelings, the real voice of my Thin Woman emerged.

April 23, 1987

I am the Thin Woman. My name is Thin Linnie. I go shopping and buy size nine dresses. Everything I try on fits and flatters. I never have to avert my eyes from the glaring dressing room mirror. No ripples nor bulges stare back at me.

I am Thin Linnie. I go to parties and pass up pastries and piles of heavy, hard-to-digest food. I choose lightness and health. I nibble raw vegetables and sip fruit juice. My mouth chooses not to be constantly chewing. I might have something interesting to say or I might want to smile at someone intriguing.

I am Thin Linnie. I bicycle for miles. My heart pumps approval. My knee appreciates the trim body it supports. Balance and grace are mine. I dance smoothly in this lightweight body.

I am Thin Linnie. You have just the slightest inkling of me now. As you bid me to appear, know that I am afraid to be, afraid to be thin, afraid of the competition of other women, afraid of the attention of men. I am terrified of attracting the wrong man.

I remember the last time I was thin. I thought it might help with my reconciliation. I wanted so to make my marriage work. Instead, it worked just the opposite. He never worried that I'd attract other men when I was fat.

I've been in hiding.
I am afraid to be.
Afraid, but I am brave.

This was one of the few entries that actually surprised me. I reread it a dozen times, amazed by the elusiveness of the obvious.

I'd always sensed that my hunger was motivated more by emotions than by bodily need. I'd even halfway understood that my scar tissue was thicker than skin. Yet, somehow I'd never made the connection between my ex-husband's mistrust and the fact that I was at the time newly svelte and sexy.

Too svelte and sexy for my own good! Or so said my subconscious mind.

Seven years later, after cutting all ties with that part of my past, I was still beating myself up for being thin!

How could this be true?

Diary Dialogue

I couldn't believe I blamed my thinness for problems with my ex-husband. I had already poured gallons of vinegar and anger into other diaries and a fistful of therapeutic poems. I couldn't possibly be blaming myself. After all, I'd rid myself of most of my bitterness toward him.

Yet, there it was in black and white. What a tangled wall of thick, thorny bushes had grown around the truth.

Lost in the emotional tangle of painful recall, I trusted my Fat Lady's courage and Thin Linnie's sincerity to lead me out of the wilderness.

Oh, I knew Thin Linnie was me. I had simply divided myself into two personnas, one fat and one thin. And in creating two separate voices, I gave myself permission to explore the trenches. To track old battle scars. To dialogue back and forth like old army buddies, reunited over a pitcher of sparkling water, a decade after going their separate ways.

March 18, 1987

THIN LINNIE: O Fat Lady, do you ever get frightened of the dark?

FAT LADY: Was it dark the night he left us?

THIN LINNIE: Dark and quiet. He didn't even say good-bye.

FAT LADY: And so you went inside and hid.

THIN LINNIE: Yes. I wanted to hide from everything that hurt me. And to grow big and bold so I wouldn't have to feel that way again.

FAT LADY: You can't keep people from leaving you. And when it hurts, you can only let the pain roll off you. Maybe that is why I came along. I am round enough to let the hurt roll off me.

THIN LINNIE: Thank you. You camouflage me well. You do not attract men the way that I did.

FAT LADY: Hush now. Let go your blame. I do not blame you for being you. Thin is innocent.

THIN LINNIE: Thank you and I do not hate you for being fat. Fat is friendly. Fat is innocent. Fat is a fine way of coping with pain and fear. Yet, we can plot a better path here in this diary. I'd like to come out and be myself. Would you help me?

FAT LADY: How?

THIN LINNIE: Oh, by finding the middle ground between us. By listening to my hopes and fears. By understanding me. By sharing your hopes and fears so that I can understand you.

FAT LADY: Yes. I can do that.

THIN LINNIE:	What are you afraid of, Fat Lady?
FAT LADY:	I'm afraid to let go of this weight. I'm afraid people won't take Toni seriously without all this bulk.
THIN LINNIE:	Why is that?
FAT LADY:	Toni fears that thin women are vainer, shallower, more preoccupied with the superficial layers of life and looks. She thinks it is what the rest of the world believes and that she knows better than to judge a book by its cover. But deep down, Toni has bought into this bigger-is-better myth.
THIN LINNIE	Isn't it?
FAT LADY:	Bigger is bigger, that's all. The kind of weight Toni wants to wield—weighty ideas and a broad viewpoint—is full of integrity and truth, not fat. I spend more time than you do worrying about how I look, wishing I were thinner. So how can I be less vain or concerned with looks than you thin women are?
THIN LINNIE:	When Toni reads this, let's tell her we both agree. We want to live a thinner, healthier, happier life.
FAT LADY:	Yes. And, Thin Linnie, let's keep talking to each other.
THIN LINNIE:	Amen.

My Fat Lady and Thin Linnie became peace keepers, no longer at odds with food. Amid a long and painful struggle, they walked the littered battlefields in search of a truce, so this war would never happen again.

I knew when I reread this entry that a true and lasting peace had finally been achieved. The treaty had many more pages to be written yet I had truly begun to think thin.

I remember a poster I had in my first apartment. It read, "Happiness—To get the real and lasting kind you have to grow it in your mind."

I grew the real and lasting kind from the inside out, as my Thin Woman emerged and came to life on the pages of my diary.

You can too.

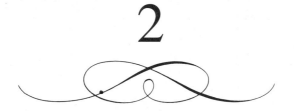

2

Getting to Like Me

Fat Chastity

To win at the game of Thinopoly, I knew I had to find all the missing pieces to Thin Linnie's fears. I had already discovered the role my physical scars played in keeping me fat, and that scars aren't always skin deep.

I also knew that understanding the unhappy resolution of my marriage was only the first step past GO. For my diary to slip me the GET OUT OF JAIL FREE card, I'd have to explore every penalty and bonus in my past love affairs.

So, I started by tracing my romantic history clear back to my juvenile crushes, analyzing every relationship in light of my diminished self-esteem. The following excerpts crystallized my insecurities so that I was able to mine them from the bedrock of my self-image, chipping away at them by using simple reason and self-acceptance.

January 30, 1987

. . . F.H. cheated on me with that thin girl. Started going steady with her, eventually marrying her. I remember crying myself to sleep, wishing I were prettier, as if thinner meant prettier . . .

February 3, 1987

. . . S.M. was so thin. I was always comparing my body to his. Instead of thinking he should gain some weight, I went around wishing I could lose 10 pounds. However, back then I really was a thin girl. Yet, because I looked at myself through his eyes, I never let myself enjoy my body. From here on in, I'm the one who defines thin . . .

February 10, 1987

. . . I'd just gotten out of casts and off crutches when I met B.C. My leg was still quite atrophied when B.C. painted a nude linear drawing of me on the wall over his bed. I never let myself believe I had inspired that piece. My leg could never provoke such bold black lines, such clean, honest art on such a grand scale.

Instead I was sure he'd done it from memory of his last woman. I never felt worthy of art or love . . .

May 23, 1987

. . . Add up the relationships, subtract the breakups. We come up with a score of nil. Love invariably leaves me hurting. Even when the end is my decision, I hurt for the other guy. When we play the role of the Fat Lady, we risk nothing. The "Big Baloney" (Hooray! A name for my Fat Lady finally emerged— "Toni Baloney" was my childhood nickname) risks nothing. For the Big Baloney, offers of love are rare.
"I guess the truth is, I am afraid to love or be loved . . ."

According to my own rule of diary writing, I wasn't ever to stop writing on a downbeat note. However, Thin Linnie had nothing encouraging to say that day. It was here that the Big Baloney became Thin Linnie's advocate.

I finished writing in the Big Baloney's voice:

May 23, 1987 (continued)

. . . I am afraid to love too. I also am afraid of rejection. I am afraid no one will ever love a fat lady. So I stay fat as a challenge to love. But love should never be double-dared into some kind of dreaded double-cross.
I know a lot about love from watching you, Thin Linnie.

You are forgetting the good things you get from loving. I know. I was on the inside watching you get all the hugs. I saw you wax and shine in love's creative glow. I listened as you wrote your best poetry. I laughed as your humor tickled the romantic comedy from the soap operas of your life.

In spite of the ending, I wish you another beginning. I wish us both another chance to soar through the heart of love, muddle through the middle. Even if we eventually end up hurting, let's let another leading man in the door.

Maybe the only reason no one will ever love a fat lady is that I won't let them.

I willingly let go of my fears. I am ready to share another chapter.

As I began to see how I was using fat to insulate myself against relationships with men, and as I began letting go of my fears and insecurities in my diary, I came to want a choice. Whether fat as a chastity belt was real or imagined, I didn't want my weight to decide my course with men.

Funny thing was, I saw losing weight as the ticket to love; however, it was while I was still 30 pounds overweight that I began dating again.

How many players does it take to win at staying thin?

Two. One Fat Lady. One Thin Woman.

And there are no losers.

Song of My Fat Self

If I was going to reinvent romance in my life, I knew I had to plot a new path to the old story of "girl meets boy."

It was the diary that allowed me to redefine relationships, from fly-by-night romance to down-to-earth, day-by-day friendship.

June 2, 1987

Okay, so I'm afraid of romance—no chance romance! Short-lived love and long-lasting heartbreak! All my affairs eventually evaporate like perfume with only a faint scent of sweetness lingering.

When there are only notions of hearts and flowers between two people, all is lost when the idealism fades. Pure romance is a capricious embrace.

However, when romance is filtered through friendship and common interests, there is a warmth that still pervades when the first flames flicker out.

Approach love like you do friendship. Passion is perishable. Friendship is a survivor's staple in the fallout shelter of love.

Although writing helps emotionally, it is action that sets change into hard physical reality. Through my diary I set goals to guide my way.

If loving myself meant befriending both my fat and thin selves, then letting someone love me meant trusting him to meet both sides of myself.

For my birthday that summer, some friends presented me with a two-month membership to a dating club. Instead of waiting until I was thin, I decided to start "as is."

If you tell yourself you are "less than" because you are "bigger than," you'll never be thin enough or good enough.

(Funny footnote to my dating diary: I never officially joined that dating club. The night of my birthday, a long-standing friendship took a romantic turn when one of the men who'd chipped in for my dating club present asked me to go dancing with him. The following summer I gave the membership to a friend who decided it was her time to dive once again into the choppy waters of romance. The thing is, the new love of my life asked me out fat and continued caring while I was thin. The point is, I realized that, fat or thin, I was the one who had barred love from my life!)

Love Is a Verb

Buckminster Fuller was the one who said that love is a verb. Bucky was a philosopher, in other words, a daydreamer, but a dreamer who knew the value of putting imagined details into solid mass. After all, he invented the geodesic dome.

I wanted to build my own dream and watch my Thin Lady become solid reality. But first I knew I had to learn to use my imagination. I did a lot of visualizing—seeing my thin woman shopping, swimming, dancing. And the more I imagined myself fit and firm, the more my behavior conspired to make it real.

Also, I found that exploring simple fantasies in my diary —size nine dresses and a moderate appetite—made me dare to dream the seemingly impossible dreams. Through the envisioning eyes of Thin Linnie, old plans and schemes emerged again and took shape as new aspirations.

As a kid, I had wanted to tour Europe by bicycle. Injury and age dissolved my trans-Atlantic hopes until Thin Linnie started describing herself as an athletic adventurer.

July 3, 1987

I am bicycling through Venice. The wind blows my hair. I outrace a gondola. My legs are tanned and muscular. The scars are there, but they mean little more than past sorrows as does the memory of being too out-of-shape to bicycle.

I love touring Europe by bike. My bicycle folds so that I ride the Eurail from country to country. I stride into the dining car and order a cup of tea and a scone.

I can enjoy pastry in moderation.

I am Thin Linnie, but not because my body is skinny, although most of my weight is, in fact, muscle. But I am Thin Linnie because my mind is lean. I carry nothing extra, no extraneous pounds nor regrets. As I soar along the colorful countryside, I know I am free to be, to feel, to do exactly as I imagine for I have designed this body, this trip, this day. I am the author of my own story, "Thin Linnie's European Bike Trek."

There are many youthful dreams that die natural deaths from lack of substance. Some of them, the silly kid stuff like my teen-age fantasy to surf the world, were better left as skeletons in the schoolyard of yesterday.

But some dreams, daring, adventuresome dreams within the stretch of possibilities, deserve to endure.

Shortly after writing the bike trek entry, I bought myself a mountain bicycle. Now, after years of bicycling, I see that it doesn't really matter if I make that trip through Europe or not. The appeal of my European fantasy was and still is wind through my hair, muscles pushing pedals, and scenery whizzing by.

Riding the bike paths of my hometown nurtured more than just a fantasy. That bike became a very important part of rehabilitating my body, grown flabby from inactivity. And what better way for a fat lady with a trick knee—and dreams of biking through Europe—to whittle down her hips.

Love is a verb.

I began to love my body enough to put my words into action.

The Feminist Mistake

All during my weight-loss process and especially once I began my Thinkercise workshops, certain feminist friends and acquaintances questioned my need to be "this thin." I looked good enough to them (and to myself); yet I kept thinking that I deserved to weigh less. However satisfied I was becoming with my rewritten self-image, I still wanted to be as lean as possible.

Yet, I was feminist enough to be concerned that my desire for leanness furthered the oppression of women, forced to slim down to the Fascist dictates of fashion trends and male preferences.

One trip through the grocery store, lugging a twenty-pound bag of potatoes assured me that my knee thrived on less weight and that health *was* indeed my primary motivation; still, I had to admit that vanity also inspired my quest.

For a while I pushed these undefined feelings aside, even though my body seemed to be stuck at my current weight. Up until this point I hadn't really been dieting. Rather I cut back on snacks, especially fats and refined carbohydrates. However, the more I reflected upon the feminist perspective of thin, the less disciplined my diet became. Not only was I not getting any thinner, I was also beginning to gain back the weight I'd lost.

As yet I hadn't really recognized the cause of my backsliding.

Then, something happened which forced me to weigh my feminist values against my desire to be thin.

At the request of a few friends, I'd been giving informal workshops in my home, sharing my journal-writing and weight-loss techniques. I'd been considering promoting those workshops on a larger scale and had applied for space at a women's center. Their reaction to my program, "Think Yourself Thin," made it impossible for me to ignore my own feminist weights and measurements any longer.

Thin is as much a feminist issue as fat.

That I preferred thin over fat did not make me a bad feminist, but I felt about as liberated as a beauty queen. I needed to give myself permission to pursue my weight goals by understanding my own pride and prejudice. My diary became a gold nugget for balancing the scales.

Moreover, my writing freed me to be thin according to my personal standards. In other words, I came to the conclusion that my thin body is healthier and more attractive than my fat one, but that does not necessarily mean that all bodies are better thin, simply that mine is.

Thin, thus, became a valid value.

And I gave myself permission to be this valuable!

February 4, 1988

What is wrong with wanting to carry the least amount of fat possible? Why do I feel guilty? I'm a bad feminist because I'm thin, as if a good one should be fat. Isn't feminism about choice? I choose being slim as a worthy goal. What's wrong with that?

The head of that women's center acted as if thin was more dirty laundry we women were being forced to wash. Maybe lean is a better term than thin; however I don't wish to rename my workshops, "Leanercises: How to Think Yourself Lean"! Nor, as she intimated, do I want to focus my life or my work on "Staying Fat and Loving It"!

As-is self-acceptance is a worthy goal. However, I believe that journal writing, as I present it, does promote the kind of self-respect that encourages as-is acceptance while at the same time presenting the opportunity for change. Furthermore, if self-acceptance is the writer's only theme and plot, then diary writing can deliver the goods; however, I choose to focus on weight loss—weight loss as a means to freedom, weight loss in the context of emotional weight first, physical weight second. Weight loss as a worthy conclusion.

I feel guilty and angry—angry because the feminist movement wasn't intended to limit, but to expand our possibilities.

That director said that by promoting weight loss I am supporting the male "woman as sex object" myth. That's unfortunate, if true; however, many good prescriptions for better health have potential negative side effects. I accept the responsibility for featuring thinness in a balanced light and dimming the focus on the sex object myth.

By promoting this emotionally healthy path to thinness, I choose to free myself and others from the feminine pursuit of perfection. I want to deemphasize food as the main ingredient in our nurturing natures. I wish to hold up a mirror to the fat that is inside and provide writing exercises, writercises, to work off the emotional flab and firm up the self-image.

I want guilt-free thinness.

How Do I Love Me? Let Me Count the Nutrients!

That last entry, and many others like it, lifted the burden I had felt from my shoulders. If others wanted to judge me guilty of vanity and vulgarity and label me a thorn on the feminist rose, the proof of my intent could be found on the pages of my diary.

I felt innocent of malice and free to court my thinness with poetry and song and a heart-shaped box of frozen grapes. I even felt free enough to begin a food diary.

I'd always avoided tracking my intake of food, because I wished instead to concentrate on the feelings I was putting into my emotional stomach. Yet, if I was serious about getting my body to its healthiest point of leanness—and I was—I knew I had to get serious about food as well as feelings.

Thus, for a full month, along with recording my daily weight I also wrote down everything I ate and why I ate it. I kept track of the nutrients I fed myself, but also the feelings inspired by certain kinds of foods.

As anyone with a junk food habit knows, there's more to eating healthy food than merely knowing an apple is a better choice than an apple tart. Emotions stand between knowing and doing, and more often than not, those emotions love to be pampered and soothed with sugar and salt, fried and buttered foods.

For example, while I was trying to lose that last 20 pounds, I worked for a small newspaper. Once a week, on production day, management rewarded our efforts with doughnuts. Ever since I worked a stint at college on the graveyard shift of a doughnut shop, those little circles of dough have been deadly enemies. One bite and my emotional appetite declared war on every rational defense I could muster. Usually I could resist the aroma and the sight of the gooey sugar and cinnamon glaze as I entered the battle zone. However, I often felt deprived when all around me, doughnuts were being dipped into coffee, disappearing with lip-licking aplomb.

In my diary I asked myself:

April 4, 1988

Would I feel bereft if I was the only non-smoker in a roomful of cancer-puffing smokers? It's basically the same thing. I'm in the minority if I choose a healthy lifestyle—a minority of winners!

Winners know their physical well-being depends upon more than the food they eat, or even their feelings or thoughts. As a trinity of body, mind, and emotions, a successful lifestyle change embraces all three.

And winners make plans and set goals. A daily agenda for a person's food intake results in pounds lost and health gained, just as surely as a business flow chart plans a corporation's path to financial reward.

I am a winner who chooses crisp apples over gooey doughnuts and takes another bite up the ladder of success toward my personal thin and healthy goals.

This and other similar entries defused my desire to be part of the coffee 'n' doughnut crew. Also, I explored the underlying alienation I felt.

April 4, 1988

It's difficult to stand apart. Yet, perhaps standing alone is the first step taken by a leader. When I know the right direction, how can I follow the crowd? I'm so used to being a little sister, taking the road well traveled, that I'm afraid to look for a new path through the woods. But the other sisters have grown fat and lazy. I can be the big sister by befriending natural sugar and refusing the empty calories of doughnuts, accepting instead the full, nutritious, content of an apple.

Those doughnuts became merely shadowy temptations. But I hadn't fully banished my junk food cravings, as I found out months later when my employer brought a cookie, candy and chip box to the lunchroom. Every time I passed that box, colorful wrappers winked up at me. At my desk, images of chocolate in her various guises would try to ambush my good intentions.

I began writing down every urge I had to make that trip downstairs and more importantly, how I was feeling immediately before and after giving in to those urgent surges for sugar.

I was hot for that junk until I poured buckets of words on the fire of my desire and finally broke the spell. Now, I am amazed by how little attraction those rows of "juju junk" hold for me at the grocery checkout line.

But for weeks, that junk box had me writing my heart out. Usually one or two sentences was enough to dissuade me. However, sometimes even the writing didn't stop me, as in the following entries:

1. I couldn't sell an ad to the publisher today. I feel dull and uncreative. I want my taste buds to have some fun with some colorful candy.
2. The receptionist is munching on a Butterfinger candy bar. I want some chocolate too.
3. My face looks tired and unattractive. I want to cry. I want some sweet chocolate.
4. I don't care what I write. This time I'm going to get some M&Ms. I deserve a decent job with a decent salary.
5. The other salesman just said my eyes never twinkle. He pretended he was joking, but I know he means it. Maybe if I eat a Twinkie my eyes will twinkle.

I was always careful not to write "I need." Telling my subconscious mind that candy is a necessity would have created a real need. On the other hand, by writing "I want," I was admitting to a true desire. That way, one truth could be countered with another, and then I had a genuine choice to make, i.e., "I want that candy but I want to be thin and healthy even more."

I wrote dozens of entries like those above, countering my feelings with thoughts about food I wanted to eat. In the beginning I occasionally relented, but soon the urges became less frequent and more easily dispelled. The above entries represent times I gave in. After nibbling, I listed the culprits in the food-intake section of my diary and wrote a *few* lines on my post-sugar feelings.

1. SNACK: 20 M&Ms
FEELING: I don't feel any more creative or able to make a sale. If that was my motive, candy didn't do the trick.

2. SNACK: Butterfinger
FEELING: So, like K., I had my chocolate fix. I felt deprived watching her have hers. Now we can both feel bloated and unhealthy together. Isn't that foolish? Anyway, I forgive my weak foolishness. Tomorrow is a day of better choices!

3. SNACK: a bag of M&Ms
FEELING: I still feel like crying. Candy doesn't change that! Junk food just makes my face look more tired and unattractive. I remember buying candy on the way to school in the eighth grade. I was always comparing myself to other girls in the class and inevitably I came up a little "less than." But the candy I bought and smuggled into class gave me the power to comfort myself, something I couldn't find in a mirror.

I was cute enough back then I could have used mirrors to focus on my attractive points instead of dwelling on my flaws. I still can. Maybe my face looks tired, but my smile can look bright if I let myself feel it. Tonight I'll give myself a facial and a healthy, happy supper.

4. SNACK: chocolate chip cookies
FEELING: I'm good at what I do. It would be nice to make better money, but for now I like this job. Cookies go back to the times my father would bring them home from the bakery. We were always restricted to one or two.

Cookies take me back to the holiday ones my mother would bake and hide until Christmas. Often I'd hunt them down and stuff them away. Maybe those forbidden, restricted cookies remind me of the forbidden decent wage, the restrictions created by underpaid employment. However, I know that my job and my snacks are only similar through childlike associations. I am a woman now, a woman deserving a decent salary. Cookies are not going to get me a raise. I let go the illusion of cookie comfort.

5. SNACK: Twinkies
FEELING: Those Twinkies didn't make my eyes twinkle nor my self-consciousness go away. I'm always afraid men don't see a twinkle of intelligence or humor or something special in my eyes. But that salesman was referring to surface beauty. Why should I care about shallow evaluations? It's just my insecurity, and junk won't make that go away. Twinkies can only make me fatter and less confident.

I see a twinkle of hope, of kindness, of wit and wonder in my own eyes, even if no one else does. Next time someone says something critical, I'll try to look myself in the eye and see those things there. Twinkies are for people filled with artificial cream and no surprises inside.

Over and over again, my diary let me challenge my choices. Recording what I ate as well as the feelings inspired by those particular food choices encouraged me to let go of certain fantasies I held about food. Junk food became less appealing in my mind's eye.

I never even noticed the day I quit indulging in the junk box.

My craving died of natural causes—unloved and unmourned.

The Nitty-Gritty Diet

A food-intake diary can be more than a whipping post for bad choices. A well-kept food-intake diary can be a monument to celebrate and elevate good food choices.

By recording every meal, especially friendly food— nutrient-packed, low-fat foods—my journal reinforced correct choices, choices that strengthened the Thin Woman.

Also, by recording everything I put into my mouth, I eliminated unconscious grazing. At the end of a month, certain patterns appeared in the quality and quantity of the foods I chose. The more often I snacked on fruit, the less likely cookies or other junk would appear.

Here is a typical error-free day:

June 18, 1988

BREAKFAST: 1/2 cup low-cal yogurt, 1 cup fresh strawberries, 2 tablespoons cereal, coffee
FEELING: I love this good, no-guilt, freedom feeling.

SNACK: Orange
FEELING: I feel as strong as sunshine, as colorful as an orchard.
LUNCH: Large salad with 2-1/2 ounces crab meat (canned, with the salt rinsed off), oil and vinegar dressing, 1/2 bagel (dry, no butter)
FEELING: I feel so energetic I could run a mile in the sand.
SNACK: Hard-boiled egg, chopped with chili powder
FEELING: No longer as fragile as Humpty Dumpty, I have no reason to fear a great fall.
SUPPER: One cup spaghetti squash, fresh tomato sauce with herbs, ground turkey meatballs, salad with oil and vinegar, melon
FEELING: Wow! If I am what I eat, then I am organically healthy. I feel thin enough to squeeze through the holes of a colander. As mellow as a melon. Thanks to me!
SNACK: Apple
FEELING: An apple a day keeps the cookie cravings at bay!

Since I also had begun weighing myself every day and listing the type and length of my exercising, I was able to chart the most efficient combinations for weight loss. I designed a diet plan that coordinated my appetite with my metabolism.

For a month I kept this record until I was able to whittle my diet down to a nitty-gritty, basic plan calculated so I could lose as much weight as possible and still stay healthy.

I figured I needed six to eight ounces of low-fat protein, two to three servings of fruit and the same amount of vegetables, two to three whole-grain choices, and two eight-ounce servings of low-cal dairy products.

I drank lots and lots of water. I began drinking eight to ten glasses of water and taking a B complex for stress and a good C vitamin for basic health.

Only when I ate something off-diet did I write about my food feelings.

Yes, it took a lot of energy to devise my own Nitty-Gritty Diet, yet it has become a lifetime plan for healthy eating.

Still Life

I sat on a big boulder of an apple
under a banana moon
in a broccoli grove
watching the river of rice flow,
wondering how I ever lost my way.

Seems I'd been wandering in the dark chocolate,
stumbling over jelly beans and licorice logs,
stuck in quicksand of chicken fat,
for longer than it takes
fudged arteries to harden into a soft ball.

And while I sat and stewed,
it started sprinkling parsley flakes
while winds of garlic stirred
my cauldron of confusion
into an aromatic broth.

I wept to think of all the refinement,
the energy gone into processing
and packaging and persuading me
that the red dye of an M&M
was purer than a radish or a beet.

And yet, as the lemon sun rose
I saw the road to wellness
paved in paper and paprika—
natural recipes bridging me past
monosodium's better glutamate.

Mind-flexing

Phil Donahue once did a show about anorexia nervosa. He interviewed the parents of a young woman who had died of a heart attack brought on by severe malnutrition. Her disease seemed to have been triggered by a comment some young man made about her "big behind." Unfortunately, the perfectionist in her took the comment to heart and quit eating.

Absurd behavior? Ridiculous reaction? Eccentric and strange?

Maybe. Maybe not.

I have often tried to change my appearance based upon someone else's opinion. I too have taken casual, but critical, comments to heart. Instead of starving myself, I'd try to store six months' worth of nurturing into my fat cells.

Moreover, fashion models and television stars embody images of the ultimate woman based on someone else's standards. I hadn't invented the Cosmo Girl, yet I thought I had to at least try to look like one. Those long, leggy bodies may be beyond my genetic code of possibilities, still I anguished over my bulky calves, my thick thighs. I knew I needed to stop comparing myself to these illusive icons of our society, which, liberated or not, was not an easy accomplishment when those symbols are constantly parading around in the uniform of success.

For many years, I couldn't look in a full-length mirror without dwelling on my imperfections. Instead of viewing my whole body and appreciating the symmetry of my general shape, I would focus on the dissymmetry of my legs. Instead of admiring my Scarlet O'Hara-slim waist, I dwelled on my Hattie-fattie hips.

I deserved better. And I found it in my own reflection.

Mirror, mirror in my mind, I'm just as fair as any I can find.

I wrote up some mirror-etiquette rules and taped them to my full-length mirror. They stayed there until they became second nature.

September 12, 1988

1. I will always find something nice to think about my image.
2. I will respect my own shape without bogus *Vogue* expectations.
3. I will look in my own eyes for the inner beauty that truly matters.

Once I read an article in a popular women's magazine about how women distort their own proportions. Using outstretched hands, a number of women estimated the width of their hips. Not surprisingly, a significant majority of women overstated their girth.

Of course, I was right up there with the worst of the overestimators. That encouraged me to begin to put a new slant on my mirror and encouraging words in my vocabulary.

July 6, 1988

You're looking really good, Thin Lady. More than mere thinness, you have a healthy glow about you. All those vegetables and fruits, helping your hair shine and your eyes twinkle. (Yes, they do twinkle.) When I see other women who are my size, I don't see them in the harsh light I evaluate myself. Viewing my own body with the same kind eyes I afford friends and strangers would be a good, new step for me.

August 3, 1988

I like the muscle definition that's returning to my arms. All those arm twister exercises are really paying off. My hips are still full and that's all right. My full-bodied figure represents the average woman. All those ultra-slim magazine models account for less than 1 percent of womanly figures. That means I can see my hips as normal.

By continually basking in my diary light, I pumped up my own self-esteem. No need to depend on someone else to compliment my every success. I also took the advice I wrote for myself back when I was breaking the junk-box habit, that is, I began looking at the total me in the mirror and stopped dwelling on specific flaws.

Rather than building arrogance and conceit, self-encouraging words simply countered years of negative messages I'd been sending myself, both consciously and subconsciously. We all have little recorders in our brains with tapes playing constantly. I learned to erase those old tapes and record self-acceptance speeches.

The final result—I know for whom the bell tolls. It tolls for me.

Poetry in Emotion

Sometimes I got downright poetic befriending my Fat Lady and serenading my Thin Woman in the verses of therapeutic poetry or "therapoetry." I began a poem titled "Confessions of a Fat Lady" about the time I started giving workshops for friends who wanted to learn along with me to write themselves thin. I worked on that poem for about a year, editing and refining words and feelings, admiring the view of both my Fat Lady and Thin Woman.

Poetry invites the imagination along on a rhythmic ride through heartfelt feelings and mind-bending ideas, using visual images to catch the right wave to some distant shore of conclusions.

Modern poetry is a lot freer than the metered verse that may have bored you back in English Composition 101. Throw out the rules of grammar and syntax. My only criterion for calling something poetry is that it's written down.

"Therapoetry" is just what it sounds like—the poetic tension release of therapy plus the therapeutic calm of poetry. Which comes first—the therapeutic or poetic intent? Generally, they evolve simultaneously. Sitting down to write is therapeutic in itself. When you play with words to express your feelings in a compressed way, often your feelings change as you edit and alter your therapoetry.

I have read my "Confessions of a Fat Lady" at numerous poetry gatherings and never fail to receive diverse reactions, including one woman's lament that it took her appetite away!

confessions of a fat lady

Bless me Butterbud for I have sinned
I lied to my brothers
stole from my sisters
disobeyed my parents
and worst of all—
I got fat

"Never get FAT!"
"Never ever get FAT!"
my mother said it as if fat
was something you got from a toilet seat
as if black-netted-stilettoed women
got paid to get FAT
as if not getting fat
were worthy of college credit
a freshman prerequisite
for a career in Staying Thin
"Never Get FAT!"
—the first commandment for teen-age girls,
the zero hour for mid-life ladies!
the over-the-hill death toll.

Never get fat

my mother said it over a pile of meatballs
as if food had nothing to do with fat
as if by slanting her thin mirrors backwards
the carnival image would protect me from fat . . .
so I could eat more meatballs

Get fat?
never!
I've seen the colander's gleam
in the eyes of men
who would strain me
thinner than my mother's spaghetti
I've seen the reflective glint in women who prefer
my mother's slanted mirror
I feel my fifth grade hips
pushing out pink pleats,
pleading
"Never ever get fat!"

confessions of a dream eater

and yet, despite the slim conspiracy
I sometimes "got fat"
sometimes it happened overnight
I'd go to bed thin and dream my fat dreams
fat ladies spinning their polka-dotted mu'umu'us
legs like honey-dipped crullers
dunking into my mocha malted milk
drip, drip into June Taylor dancers
fan their taffy thighs
dribble their basketball breasts
into a hypnotic kaleidoscope
jiggling me into the
eye

inside
caterpillars
trade the metamorphosis of butterflies
for the metabolism of butterballs
all for a little padding
insulation against fat chances and slim pickings
the ultimate chastity belt
the antidote for invisibility
all while greasy mantras chant
"You're only as fat as your last meal"
"The fatter I get the freer I feel!"

in my dreams
I scale the pounds
from my rock-bottom weight
I eat myself raw
and wake up fat!

confessions of a throw-up artist

"The last spoonful always makes me fat,"
the woman who models lingerie at lunches
for businessmen, more horny than hungry,
said over her last bite
before disappearing
dental floss in hand
as if plaque was all she planned to purge
as if her building blocks weren't half-mad
for a crust or a crumb

She says "there is too much
for so little
and too little for so much"
I say "tsk, tsk, true, true"
and order another chocolate camisole

once a split-up
bequeathed me our fold-down sofa
old food stains
exiled me to softer places
tracing puckers and ruffles
when somehow I got lost in the foam—
and ate the whole thing
I'd only meant to nibble it down to a loveseat

yet upholstery loses its flavor
on the sofabed overnight
and so too did I
look a bit too comfortable
people began sitting on me
tucking their dirty underwear in my folds
and dropping loose change in my crevices
I had to do something . . .
"tsk, tsk, true, true"
and so I stuck two lamps down my throat
and up came the couch in easy-chair chunks
lopsided, one-sided comfort

after that, filling my empty frame
with still-life stuff became as easy as having it
and eating it too
days later I downed my rag rug
only to throw up in circles
of need and hunger
hunger and need
I gorged on the encyclopedias
a starving fantasizer hungry for facts
feasting on Freud's second-hand dementia
and upchucking sarong after sarong
after sarong.

celebration of a word relisher

I wish I could eat the stove
and the things that burn holes
in the things I leave too close
I wish I could eat my daughter
to save her from devouring herself
I wish I could free my mother
from meatballs and mirrors

yet I no longer chew my leg off
to free it from hunger's trap
now I eat my words . . .
every morning when fat cells
float like cereal
on the surface of last night's dream
I break the cellulite wrapper
and eat the blubber of lard-ass
adjectives from my vocabulary
and I blow beautiful bubbles
in my own bowl
and listen to the tinsel of thin
and smell the sweat in svelte
and watch the fat between my ears
dissolve
mixed and mingled
with the delicious saliva
and the sweet sentiment
of self-relish.

3

Suddenly I'm Light and Breezy

Count Down, Blast Off!

Self-relish!

Now there's a condiment that, spread evenly and honestly, enhances any "self-esteemwich."

As for my own array of personal seasonings, there was enough self-relish that very soon inner visions of my Thin Lady became as real as the outer reflection in my full-length mirror.

The new year rolled in and I was still over 15 pounds from my target weight. My goal hadn't budged and yet long before I got even close, I came to actually see and feel myself, truly believe myself to be thin (defined as lean and healthy). And because of this *imagined* thinness, I was comfortable, natural, and happy with my outer body exactly as it was then. I still intended improvement, but my desire for actual thinness did not interfere with self-acceptance and a shift into my Thin Lady's consciousness.

Like a persona in a poem, Thinness lived mostly in my imagination. Yet, for months Thinness had been trickling into the reality side of my brain.

As a result, this mental state of being thin, that is, comfortably lean and healthy in my mind, soon made the leap from thought to action. I thought of myself as thin and then began to see myself as thin in the full-length mirror in my bedroom. I still weighed well above my goal, yet the extra pounds didn't stop me from seeing "thin."

In the past, I'd reshaped my body a few times without trying. Once, after spending a long, healthy season living on a beach in Mexico, I came home weighing less than I had in years. Another time I lost a lot of weight in the name of love, but nevertheless I thought and felt fat. Too many basic, negative body beliefs were buried beneath the layers of my skin. My body hangups waited in the shadows like a drug dealer, hoping to convince me that I still wasn't good enough to live inside this healthy body. Always before, these body hangups had convinced me that I shouldn't enjoy my successful weight loss and newly improved eating habits, and that I couldn't possibly believe in this lighter version of myself.

And always before I reverted back to ice cream and cookies and lying around depressed and full of self-pity.

Perhaps as many as six other times I'd trim down 5 or 10 pounds and stop short of my desired destination. Frustration, boredom or the same old body hangups usually derailed my diet.

Now, thirteen months into keeping my weight-loss log, delays had me wondering if I'd ever drop my last few pounds.

Week after week, I went up and down like a roller coaster. Sometimes I felt permanently doomed to a kind of carnival ride for Fat Ladies. Even so, somehow I felt certain that, with the help of writing, I would eventually get off and actually be able to write myself a new kind of ride, this one designed for Thin Linnie. Why? Because this time I was weighing more than just my body on the bathroom scale. This time I was charting my emotional weight and dropping unnecessary pounds between the lines of my diary. This time I was consciously, carefully aware of what was going through my mind and into my mouth. This time the choices belonged to me.

And so, determined to carry a more balanced proportion of body fat and lean muscle, I began to write to each and every pound I intended to lose.

March 2, 1987

What happened? I'm up to last week's weight again!

I've been depressed and you didn't come to cheer me with bouquets of words planted on white fields of paper. You've been avoiding the pen just when I needed it most. You have a twenty-four-hour, on-call therapist and yet you try to hide your thoughts and emotions behind something from the refrigerator.

You've been feeding your stomach as if it were insatiable, instead of nurturing your hungry heart.

You come home mid-afternoons to write, but instead you prowl the empty house feeling alone and abandoned. Steven, my dear and beloved friend, isn't going away for another two months and already you feel deserted. You feel alone. Okay. But is food going to make his leaving any less painful? Remember back when you accepted love with all its consequences?

Now you're feeling sorry for yourself, wishing to turn back the heart as if it were time, time that can only be taken on its own terms, minute by minute.

Minute by minute and pound for pound.

I want to be a pound less than I weigh now. I want to be a woman who does not drown in food. I want to be a slim woman who can let go of love and pounds without regret.

It was true, Steven made a decision to move to San Francisco in order to be closer to the art scene, and I was allowing myself to wallow in self-pity and self-recriminations. Even though his actual departure was months away, I was already dreading the approaching lion of loneliness. So, I munched through the tangled jungle of my feelings, snapping potato chips underfoot.

I knew that I was overeating by choice, especially since writing could save me. Experience had shown me that if I wrote regularly, suppressed emotions would not sabotage my story. However, I was acting like an obstinate child who refuses to open her mouth for medicine, even if it was cherry-flavored syrup and would help what ails me.

Often I had to force my own hand.

Fortunately, diary writing works magic even for the reluctant-hearted. Now that I think back to my youthful diaries, the ones I bemoaned earlier in the introduction, I see how even those discouraging words, that constant outpouring of pessimism and doubt, helped heal me. For the creative process is inherently healing. As for those last few pounds, I kept at my writing, every day, counting down the pounds and letting go more fears until I broke through to my personal best, my individual thin winning line.

March 13, 1987

The scale stays stable and so do I. I can visit Steven when he leaves. Meanwhile, I am now the Thin Linnie who believes she'll soon be one pound less. She is just taking an extra day or two to do it.

Since breads are my weakness, I'll have my allotted last piece at the end of my day—as a treat. A treat worth waiting for.

I know my desire for bread is connected to Steven's leaving. Yet, seeking comfort in starch is a mistake, one I learned from all the bakery goods Daddy brought home and the treats Mommie baked. Yes, it was an expression of my parents' love, but it is not the kind of love that helps. Maybe sweet pastries comforted me as a skinny kid, but sweet, starchy, white flour and sugar is not comfortable when it turns into fat. Think of it as the same stuff that stiffens collars. Do I really want to be a stuffed shirt? Think of cakes and cookies as cornstarch, a food thickener and filler. Think of butter and lard as pure vegetable and animal fat. Is that what I really want to be?

All the pretty pastries in the world will not fill up the void left by Steven, nor thicken me to better withstand the hurt. Steven brought me to new understandings of myself, new horizons of romantic relationships, and new heights (plus assorted lows) for loving.

I always knew Steven was not "the one," the "one" being a man compatible enough to last a lifetime. What if, for me, there is no "one"? What if, for me, there is only the alternative, that is, loving "the many"? What if . . . what if?

I've been raised to view loving more than "the one" as romantic failure. On the contrary, perhaps I am naturally drawn to several because there are many branches of my own tree of love that need tender attention. And maybe my ever-loving tree was not intended to be straight and narrow, but to grow and explore the fullness of loving "the many." Someday I may meet that rest-of-my-life partner, that nearly perfect soul mate. But, hasn't every man I've loved thus far been a partner in my life?

If I see Steven as another tree whose branches twined and grew with mine for a while, perhaps this time of separation will be healthier and happier for both of us.

As untraditional as it sounds, maybe my love lines were meant to continually add and subtract. Nevertheless, if I hadn't drawn out my feelings in my diary, I probably would have missed the opportunity to appreciate "the many," and felt like a failure because I hadn't found the praised and precious "one."

Self-analysis is so simple, so logical, and yet so healing.

Putting my feelings on paper made me feel better and kept me from calories, but what about my daughter Jessica? What kind of role-model mother was I being for her?

March 15, 1987

Okay, so what is wrong with loving more than one man? I guess I fear putting Jessica on the wrong road —as if there were only one straight and narrow highway. As much of a nonconformist as I am, I still want traditionalism for her, but only because a rebel's way is rougher. I want her life easier than mine. And yet, how vain to think I could or should decide her fate! All I can do is to live my love honestly and teach her to follow her own heart wherever it leads.

For some, like me, that has meant loving several men. Jessica will be exposed to the pursuit of one everlasting love through the example of my sisters and their husbands. I cannot control which way she herself chooses. It is vain to think I have that kind of power and control even over an only daughter. Okay, so here and now I let go my illusions of control.

What else is wrong with loving more than one man?

I think I fear it is a watered-down version of true love. Well, maybe for some people it is, but for others it isn't. Why can't love be transferable? If I reach a certain depth in the love I feel for someone, and then the one I love leaves, I can choose to transfer the power and the beauty of it elsewhere. Love is only watered down if I let it be.

Also, love has matured for me. Love has different faces, different lifestyles. Okay, so again I let go the "one and only" notion. What else do I fear? I fear hurting Jessica's self-esteem. I fear Steven's leaving will tell her something about herself—that she is not good enough or he would stay. But isn't that a transference of my own fear? It *is* true that Jess will probably believe whatever it is I believe about his leaving. If I believe he is leaving because I am not good enough, then she will adopt my definition for loving and leaving for herself. Yet, if I project the unemotional, objective truth—that we are not compatible enough to stay together in this intense relationship and that he should pursue his art

wherever his heart leads, then she will trust her
friendship with him. And the more she will trust me.
Also, the more balance I can maintain while letting
Steven go, the more Jessica will embrace his fatherly
love for her and I will have his friendship in place of
his romantic love.

Remember this, the next time I become
emotionally overdramatic.

And so on. More than simply working on my weight
issues, my diary explored the heavy issues of my life. My
still-life self-portraits recorded internal changes as they occurred
and allowed me to fully integrate them emotionally.

Writing from the deep recesses of myself exposed the
many obstacles on my path to thinness. By exploring my hopes
for love and fears of its demise, I was able to pursue the other
loss—the shedding of pounds.

March 19, 1987

. . . still waiting for Thin Linnie to reach the finish
line, weight-wise. Maybe tomorrow. I am not losing a
Fat Lady, I am gaining a big beautiful inner light. I am
not losing love, I am gaining the opportunity to
redefine it . . .

And even when my scale failed to show any physical
changes, I continued to serenade myself. I continued to believe
in Thin Linnie.

I wrote her like I would any fictional character; that is,
I allowed her to express her feelings freely. Moreover, like any

character created with imagination and inspiration, Thin Linnie could not help but become more and more real with every word.

March 22, 1987

Congratulations, one-pound-lighter Thin Linnie, but who are *you*? I am you, changing into an emotionally and physically thinner lady. I like jogging on the trampoline while watching the "Oprah Winfrey Show." I haven't exercised for a few weeks. Today I begin again.

Every day I wrote, and each day I felt more certain that letting go of incompatible love would help me to let go of uncomfortable weight.

April 2, 1987

I am Thin Linnie no matter what I weigh. I am the same person as I will be when I lose another pound.
 Steven leaves June 1. Lots of time to let go. I do not need food for comfort now, nor when he goes. Just like a body grown too large for comfort's sake, our relationship has grown too uncomfortable for our individual growth. We became weighed down in each other's definitions of ourselves. I will miss Steven dearly, yet I know how to enjoy my solitude . . .

And so on, until a week later.

April 9, 1987

The scale has said the same for the fourth day in a
row. Hurrah! Yet I know I really weigh 2 pounds less.
I feel good now and I will feel good when those last 2
pounds are gone. I'm not afraid to weigh less—I like
it. I think my fear is of being alone and that it relates
to my fear of death. Aloneness is as inevitable as
death, but solitude is also open to almost unlimited
possibilities. Think of this—when I spent all that time
alone during the surgeries, I finished three drafts of a
novel. With Steven, I haven't been able to finish one
draft of the new novel.

Who knows where solitude (death?) will take
me and so why worry? Solitude leaves space for
creativity and, yes, even time for new people to enter
my life.

The more I contemplated the quiet grace of solitude
which would come with Steven's passing, the less I viewed our
separation with desperation. I seemed to shed a pound of fat with
every pound of fear.

And I continued dropping pounds and fears until I finally
reached a snag. For two weeks my weight zigzagged up and
down 3 pounds. Every time my weight went down, my eating
became erratic and compulsive, settling back down only when
I'd gained back those pounds over and over again.

By posing the question in my diary, "What's wrong with
weighing the weight I want?" I finally tied the loose ends into a
neat knot that, on the surface, seemed to have little to do with
my present predicament.

I wrote the following midway through a quart of yogurt
—at least the quality of my binge food was improving.

April 24, 1987

I want to weigh less, but if I keep eating that yogurt, I'll be back up again before I can stir the fruit up from the bottom. I feel fat already. At least Steven doesn't like yogurt and won't get mad if there's none left. He hates when I drink the last of the milk.

I remember baking a cake once and nibbling throughout the day, so that by late afternoon I'd eaten half the cake. Then, when I thought of my ex-husband coming home and ridiculing me, I ate the rest of it. Why I didn't just cut up the cake and pretend it was baked in a smaller pan, I don't know. I was so crazy back then, trying to cure his sadness and defuse his hostility. I had to hide all evidence of my gluttony. It might make him unhappy or angry.

Back then I weighed less than I do now! I wonder if I'm afraid to weigh what I did during those heartbreaking days? What am I trying to hide now? Now, on the brink of Steven's departure, the two passages feel somewhat similar, at least in that they both hurt. I'm trying to paint over the teardrops with fruit smudges and yogurt smears. I forgive my weakness and remember that I don't need food to cope. After my ex-husband was gone, there were years of being alone, not dating, not socializing. I needed that kind of seclusion back then. I don't need it now. If that's what I'm afraid of, I don't need to worry.

These strokes down memory lane cleared out the blocks on my path, allowing me to continue calming down my fears and walking off my pounds.

Most of the time I could plow through the rubble with prosaic ease. Occasionally I needed a bulldozer and would have to dig for hours.

Thank God the shovel I needed was as light as a feather pen. And on my daughter's birthday my pen revealed to me a secret I never dreamed possible.

May 23, 1989

Happy birthday, baby! What a birthday for us both, Jessica. Today you're ten and today I have lost another 5 pounds!

You've reached a milestone, my dear, for you have turned ten with your kind, gentle nature intact, even though so many children have ridiculed you for your one white eye. I am proud of you! I hope you let yourself feel pride in your accomplishment.

I am proud of me too! I have worked hard to become Thin Linnie, just 4 pounds short of my original goal. I kept feeling thin enough, but that my target weight kept repeating itself in my mind. You know something, Jessica, my present weight is just right. I have reached my goal. And no I'm not settling for less —or in this case, more. Whether or not I ever lose another pound, I am now the Thin Woman I wish to be.

No, there are no fireworks out there. I wonder if I anticipated some? I still feel the same amount of joy as I felt yesterday, when I weighed more. My life will not be instantly marvelous. I don't want to get hung up with grandiose expectations. I still have bills to pay and wrinkles to worry about.

Ah, the wrinkles. Suddenly I'm an older woman, a middle-aged mother. I guess that's something I'll need to work out in another notebook—the Diary of an Old Lady!

Fat or thin, baby-bottom smooth or old-lady crinkled, I am still me. I still miss my Mommie and Daddy and sisters and often wish I'd never set off to find my fortune so far from home. This new milestone does not erase the scars that mar my leg. My dresser drawers and closets are still a jumbled mess. I still need a new car, and Steven still leaves in a week. I still wish I were prettier, smarter, and had more money. Being thin doesn't magically cure all that ails me.

Being thin is just that—being thin. Thin Linnie looks better in clothes than the Big Baloney. I feel better and I know I'm healthier. It's a lot of weight off my shoulders, as well as my knees. Still I have the same day-to-day hassles to contend with and if I think thin is an instant cure for life's other ills, then disappointment will surely fatten me back up again.

I accept this new birthday of Thin Linnie as a rebirth of honesty here on the pages of my diary. I will continue to confront my fears and record my joy.

By allowing myself to reevaluate and reset my goal, I freed myself from the bondage of charts and scales. Because of my healthier, more active lifestyle, I later dropped a few more pounds—but those numbers never really mattered. Like Dorothy in Oz with her magic slippers, once I learned to believe in Thin Linnie, I was already home.

Now I had to learn to live in Kansas.

Fatal Detractions

Moreover, I had to continue walking the same road I'd been traveling, occasionally hobbling and stumbling along, for so many years. And that road was littered with fast-food hangouts, slow-to-heal hang-ups, and junk food pick-me-ups.

While my body was going through its changes, I noticed a few friends going through some changes of their own. A woman who'd been very supportive and helpful while I was convalescing from the surgery following my accident slowly became cold and critical. My first reaction accorded her little understanding.

March 10, 1987

Today V. said my face was too thin, said I looked older now that I'm thinner. Last time I saw her, she said that since slimming down, I'd become flat-chested. What's the matter with her? Why does my weight loss threaten her? She liked me better as the Big Baloney, with so little confidence I barely asserted any opinions. Perhaps V. likes me better weak because she needs to feel superior. Yet, I don't wish to just cut her out of my life—she was so kind and considerate during my surgeries. But I can't become the old weak self again and so she is the one who has a choice to make. I hope she can learn to accept this new stronger me.

Now I realize that I was angrier than this entry implied. I remembered that after my motorcycle accident I lost a few friends. It wasn't just bones that broke back then. My spirit fractured as well. I don't necessarily think the accident caused the changes, but rather the trauma confirmed my deepest self-doubts, disguised though they had been by youthful bravado. Even my personality was unrecognizable to friends who wanted to rock 'n' roll with the old me, not sulk with this saddened soul entombed in plaster.

Here was a friend who, after all these years, had on the surface rejected me for my thinner body, but who I was certain resented my self-confidence. She wanted to sulk with the saddened soul and I wanted to, if not rock 'n' roll, then bike 'n' hike.

In responding to V.'s reaction, I think I was actually mourning old losses, as well as bemoaning her conduct. It wasn't until I'd begun analyzing another friend who'd suddenly wanted to go work out at the gym together, that I realize V.'s attitude was not rooted in malice.

April 2, 1987

I know that I should take K.'s sudden interest in me as a compliment to my new self, still I feel insulted. Why didn't she come around more when I was on crutches when I really needed her?

Funny, K. likes me better strong and confident while V. liked me better weak and unsure. And I'm disappointed that either of them has a preference. I want everyone to take me as I am. Maybe only family does that—if you're lucky!

What if V., being an only child and mother of four, needs to feel needed, which she could when I was convalescing; while K., being the oldest child of a large family, didn't want someone else depending on her. Maybe I need to understand we all fulfill certain

needs for each other, and just because I change
doesn't mean other people's needs will automatically
change to match mine.

Maybe I need to be who I want and need to be,
regardless of what others want and need from me.

Read 'Em and Weep

Keeping a keen eye on my own emotions made more sense than
trying to gage and control the feelings of friends, especially since
in one more day, Steven, who knew and loved the Big Baloney,
would move away.

Steven's imminent departure stirred up all kinds of the
old feelings I'd stewed about before. Feelings of abandonment
and rejection wafted up from my overseasoned casserole of lost
loves. Thank God I'd become my own best pen pal.

May 31, 1987

I helped Steven pack and watched him load the van to
go. He leaves first thing in the morning. Why do
artistic men always leave me! Maybe I'm too
understanding, too liberating. As a striver and a
survivor, I encourage them to seek their dreams and
then fall apart when they do.

Sixteen years ago when B.C. packed his Saab
to go back to New York—also to pursue his art—I'd
been too damned darling about it until the very last
moment when all his stuff, crammed tight in the back
seat and high on the hood, stared me square in the eye.

Then it hit me in the gut, "He's taking his junk and leaving you behind!"

Oh, how I bawled! I watched him pull away and stood in the street and sobbed like a baby, screamed like a crazy woman. My dignity drained down the empty street, the muddy water of my tears catching in puddles inside the gutters of despair.

It sounds so melodramatic, but it was even worse!

God, I wanted so to go with him. Instead, I sent him a copy of Hermann Hesse's *Knulp*, a book about a vagabond loner who triumphed through his solitary wanderings.

I would have begged if I'd thought B.C. would have stayed—or better yet, taken me along. Now I see what I didn't see then.

The city wouldn't have called B.C. so many years before, as it is calling Steven now, if I was "the one" for him.

The part of me that wants Steven to stay is that same little girl from seventeen years ago who sobbed in the streets, so certain true love was driving out of my life forever. That it did and it didn't is the saving grace here.

For Steven is one of the several I have loved, leaving me to make room for another.

I can let go this love with enough dignity to keep me from groveling on the gravel driveway. I can maintain enough self-respect to keep my eating normal and healthy, to keep loving my own body enough to let myself grieve on tears and poetic loneliness, instead of cookies and milk.

Someone said we are an overstimulated society, grown accustomed to alternating our moods, if not with food, then with drugs, alcohol, gambling, love, or money. Now that I have been highly sensitized by love, I fear that I will stuff myself numb when he actually goes!

Yet, writing this, I see I have choices.

The ennui of mindless eating versus the intense reality of feeling. I own this love and thus this loss, in all its brilliant light and haunting shadow. Grieving is a necessary part of the farewell. If I accept the beginning of the grieving process, even now while he is still here with me, then I can welcome it as the beginning to the end of pain.

Love is being lost every minute that he is here. Right now I feel his loss. I weep for tomorrow. My pink-pleated little girl pounds her fists against the closing doors of emotions that leave me so wide open. So weep, little girl, and then let him go with grace and style.

Let yourself feel, not the bloat of food, but the triumph of truth. Truth is its own hearty repast. Experience your life without need of mind-altering substances. Feel even the sadness, the utter despair of losing love without retreating into a food-induced stupor.

And when he leaves, let me banish this appetite for sugar and spice and things not so nice for my body.

When the time finally came, Steven's departure was anything but easy for me. However, having explored my emotional undercurrents, I was not carried away in a tidal wave of grief, nor did I sink in sorrow when the weepy whirlpool hit.

Yes, I had a few bad days with food, but I also found myself heading more often to my desk than my refrigerator for solace.

Help! They Only Love Me for My Body!

Just because I worked out much of the insecurity that Steven's departure brought out in me, it didn't mean I could bank those secure feelings and draw interest on the balance.

Yes, I'd become much surer of who I was and where I wanted to go.

Yes, loving in the open, honest manner that we had helped me to open my mind and integrate more truth into my communications, both literary and personal. My novel-in-progress, tentatively titled, *Fat Farm Fakir*, was all the better for the time I spent with Steven and now for the time I was spending alone finishing it.

And yes, I still felt abandoned. The Big Baloney felt the rejection more than Thin Linnie did. This dichotomy of characters allowed me to separate my positive and negative emotions into a dramatic play of worried words and wonderful wisdom.

> BIG BALONEY: I should have exercised my legs more. If my thigh muscles had been tighter, he would not have been so embarrassed by our age difference. (Steven was more than a decade my junior.)
> THIN LINNIE: He may have wanted our body more if our thighs were firmer, but you would still have been at odds over the same differences.
> BIG BALONEY: Yes, I will always want more music than news in my life and he will always prefer fishing to dancing. He wants life simple and well grounded,

while I will always seek clouds and honeycomb scintilla.

THIN LINNIE: More than body barriers, it was temperamental differences that separated us. No fault, no blame.

BIG BALONEY: Yes, and nobody's shame. Still, I miss his easy smile, the earthy understanding in his dark eyes.

THIN LINNIE: But think of the new shades of color you saw by sharing his vision for a while. You can carry that bright innocence, his provocative shapes, seductive slants, and whimsical perspectives of his inner landscapes forever within your mind's eye and heart. How richly visual your words have become because you were absorbed in the wordless aura of his art.

BIG BALONEY: Ummm. Won't memory of his color and shapes fade and blur like old photos?

THIN LINNIE: And when they do, you will miss him less. Don't worry, joy will win out here. Respect will protect his image and preserve it on something like a mental videotape. Then, when we need to re-run a cherished memory or borrow a bit of his vision, we'll just hit the play button.

Oh, what freedom awaits me always, on the pages of my diary paper. Oh, how grateful I am to have discovered that relief can come so easily in writing.

Every word I wrote about letting go of love helped me a bit more to actually let go my grief and fear.

Conversations between my imaginary characters encouraged me to find the balance between my remorseful feelings of rejection and my confident understanding of necessary change. We all have more than one character inside us waiting for the right dialogue to bring them alive.

The more dialogue I wrote, the more I began to really believe that to some extent I could intentionally direct my life the way I could create a plot in a novel. The supporting evidence was that, just like any good, inspired story, my life began to follow a course natural to the new self I was continually creating and renewing.

So, a few months later, my life naturally turned once again toward romance. With Steven as a soft spot in my heart, I began dating another man.

And as settled as I thought my man-woman-weight issues were, this new pair of eyes, looking at me in the light of romance, stirred up a dust storm of old doubts. There seems to be no end to the directions the winds of love can take.

July 29, 1987

Help! He only loves me for my body!
Maybe it's silly, but I wonder if Tom would still like me if I were fat? I don't wish to test him by actually gaining back the weight, but I can't help wondering whether he likes my active ingredients or just the more attractive packaging.
Maybe I should consider whether or not I would have been attracted to him if he looked different? Maybe, maybe not. Now that I know him, would I still like him if he went bald overnight or his belly overhung his belt? Of course, I would. I might find him less physically attractive, yet I would still like him the same. So, if he would find a bigger me less appealing physically, I would still make him think and laugh and feel.

Why am I worrying now? Isn't part of wanting to lose weight wanting to be more attractive? I've gotten what I wanted. So, enjoy his lyrical heart and his scientific mind and quit looking for problems!

And so on. Doubt still lingered like an apparition in my attic, yet with my diary cleaning out the cobwebs, I could clear the dusty air of uncertainty. Also, with my pen opening the curtains and letting in shaft after shaft of light, dispersing the ghosts that hide in ignorance, I held tight to the reflection of Thin Linnie, smiling there in the old bureau mirror where once a pink-pleated little girl looked at her average body and called it fat.

And I hadn't waited until my scale verified her existence for me. I began by opening my heart and mind to Thin Linnie in much the same way I earlier embraced my Big Baloney.

I continue to look Thin Linnie in the eye, smile, and invite her to dance to the uneven music of my life.

And Thin Linnie loves dancing in the limelight.

No, I'm not as perfect as my writing may seem to imply. No, I don't always feel healthy, thin, attractive, and happy. Most of the time, yes, but not all of the time.

However, living in a thin body means more than possessing slim limbs and trim hips.

I like to compare "thinking thin" with recycling. Sorting our daily garbage is a powerful, loving act that can, and hopefully will, save our planet. Sorting through my thoughts and feelings about food and exercising my body were certainly necessary on a daily basis if I wanted to maintain my thinness.

With continued practice, I streamlined the energy and time needed to recycle my personal wasteland—both emotional and physical.

Through my diaries, I have become able to recognize and use the buried treasures of my Big Baloney's hopes and fears. Her nonbiodegradable garbage is easily dumped in my diary.

Which leaves Thin Linnie more time and space for joy!

I guess, in a way, I have become a rewritten version of myself. As with all good rewrites, my basic theme kept its original inspiration—that of seeking balance, truth, and happiness. Through all this diary writing, my style loosened up, my plot thickened, and my body thinned.

And I began to have as much fun as I hoped.

4

Day by Day

The Undulating Dance of Change

Late night and early morning hours often find me sitting with pen in hand (or at the computer), with lyricism in mind. Ordinarily, to accompany my words, I play a little music on the stereo. Sometimes it's classical Vivaldi or New Age Kitaro, but I'm just as likely to be listening to a little boogie-woogie blues, rock, or jazz. Even the sweet, screeching strains of my daughter practicing her violin can become background inspiration for my verse.

Music, especially the wordless kind, can both relax and stimulate, which is a powerful Zen state for creativity. I believe that I would not have fallen in love with words to the extent I have, had not music been closely caressing my ears and soothing me—body and soul.

And, oh, such healing is to be found in the unbridled truth of music! No wonder some of our ancestors invented muses to watch over their songs. In many premodern societies, music was at the center of everything. Whole villages came together to celebrate the human spirit and worship nature through music, dance, and song.

Medieval folks believed their faires opened doors to fairies, and that they serenaded sprites with the festivity of their music. Occasionally, even a wandering gnome or elf might be lured from the forest with lutes or lyres. Eventually, fearful that their fetes might enrage their gods and goddesses for trying to imitate divinity (and, of course, because they had to eat), these ancestors returned reluctantly to their fields and daily harnesses.

Ah, but with a song in their hearts!

Today, in certain circles those ancient rhythms are being replayed, reexplored, redefined, and finally alchemized into something called the New Age.

Furthermore, although my descriptions reflect my own earliest European roots, village gatherings centered around music are common throughout all human history, whether accompanied by African drums, Arabian cymbals, or Indian zithers.

Consider that the ancient Gaelic people believed that music predates man and that it even had a part in the very creation of living things. Or that Indonesian musicians believe music to be continuous in the universe and that players, instead of creating it, simply make audible something that has been going on soundlessly all the time. Consider that anthropologists continue to search for a culture without any music.

What does the ancient history of music have to do with the present dance of change?

As a culture, we have changed so many of the natural movements our bodies once made that dance no longer is the free expression—the poetry in motion—that once undulated through our midst in times of joy. Nevertheless, for those who listen for the music, be it on a radio or in a forest stream, music heals.

And if music heals, imagine the power and the pleasure in responding to the chords by moving your body, that is, by undulating your limbs and torso in waves to match the music. Dance. It's that simple.

Maybe music inspires me so and dance seems so natural to me because I spent so many years casted in plaster of Paris, or as I call it, plastered and casted in Paris.

Often while I'm sitting at my desk, a catchy rhythm will set my heart to dancing and my feet to tapping, and before long, I'm up jitterbugging or ballercising (balletlike movements).

Also, dance is essential to my being able to think like a thin woman. Although she's my best audience, the Big Baloney hardly ever dances. Thin Linnie, on the other hand, can hardly stand still around foot-stomping music. I wouldn't be surprised if Thin Linnie hasn't upped my metabolism, considering the way she shakes her legs underneath my desk.

Sometimes when I dance around my living room, I imagine myself a thin, willowy tree, stretching upward, limbs growing out beyond the walls. The ceiling seems to expand almost into the sky. Or if I'm lucky enough to be dancing outside, then perhaps I am a long-necked bird with muscles tight, flying through a storm of sound. Or a puppet, sometimes playfully jerky with a jazzy beat, or gracefully swaying, as the hands that hold the puppet strings interpret the music that touches my soul.

My movements begin quite deliberately until the music almost seems to flow through me. That is when I can abandon my conscious control and for a few, wonderful moments I become what I am imitating. In this way, I *am* music!

There can never be too much dance.

Or too much music.

I also become the tree or the bird. In a world where the natural landscape is so quickly painted over by spilling black oil or left empty by trees thoughtlessly felled for commercial reasons, there can never be enough empathy for birds and trees.

Whatever image comes into my body while I'm dancing, I allow it to move me. This kind of empathetic dance and abandonment of self to music balances my emotions while toning me physically.

After a few years of high-stepping to music, I was able to replace most of my boring floor exercises with dance. Sit-ups were supplanted by the stomach-tightening moves of Pee-Wee Herman's "Big Shoe Dance," and leg lifts were transformed by my one-legged, albeit lopsided, arabesque.

As a dancing fool, my spirit began to lighten and so too did my step. The stuttering limp that once dragged down my steps became less and less impeding.

As with any old war wound, my leg does ache from time to time. Although a massage and an ice pack can stimulate lagging circulation and soothe swelling, a few doses of dancing relieve the tender stiffness that goes beyond the bone. Maybe dance can't cure all life's ills or even stave off the arthritic encroachment of age. However, an occasional application of a free-spinning fandango sure gets more than just my toes tapping again.

Dancing feet got my wheels of hope turning. Like a drum roll introducing a new entry onto the stage of my life, my dancing heart thumps out hope and harmony.

Words almost sound fake when trying to describe the healing and uplifting rhythms of the solitary dance. I believe the illusory poetry in my motions and the illuminating flow of my emotions, far more splendid than my most eloquent verse.

Often when I dance, I feel the spirit of a once prolific dancer move through me, and for the briefest millisecond my limbs possess her perfect balance. For that fleeting moment I feel wings on my artificial knee, and I'm humbled when I think about Leigh Phillips, the wheelchair ballerina, the handicapped actress-choreographer of many a university campus, the dancer who lost her footing at the age of thirteen. She inspired me inside my plaster cast to dance in spite of all. Strange as it sounds, I sometimes allow her spirit to occasionally borrow my limbs, limbs which, although disfigured and imperfect, can still kick up a heel or two.

Isn't that what the love of life and the life in art is all about!

June 21, 1988

Move me, sway me, shimmy me into a *gambado*
of change, a *pachanga* of shake
boogaloo these bent and borrowed wings
beyond the crippling crest of clay feet
my hokey-pokey hopes heed the horns
harping together for this cotillion
where moonbeams dance in my mind
reeling in the empathetic line
to catch me fishtailing beyond the tide
beyond the paralyzing tremble of doubt
move me, jig me, trot me beyond the *beguine*.

Dancing in the Rain

Water. Wet, weepy, and wonderful in its natural no-cal, no need for preservatives or artificial coloring state—ah, what liquid pleasure.

Water. Everyone from Dolly Parton to my Aunt Lillian to Doctor Stillwater swears by it. It's the most abundant element on the planet and in our bodies. It puts out fires and turns soil fertile. It quenches and revives, flushes out toxins, keeps the mind flowing and the emotions afloat.

As I learned to listen to my inner tides, my need to drown myself in food evaporated. And as I began to enjoy the simple pleasure of food, more naturally prepared, I also began to drink more and more water.

Ah, water.

It's the real thing!

January 19, 1988

Water, oh, water. How do I love thee—let me count the glasses. Day by day.

One glass keeps the Twinkies and Ding-Dongs at bay.

The second one flushes fat down the drain while refreshing my brain.

A third keeps knees and elbows from creaking and a fourth keeps my appetite from sneaking up and dragging me into the mid-day weakening of wanton grazing.

That fourth water chaser wakes me up for a fifth.

And the headwaters of that sixth glass floods
out all doubt that lucky seven will roll me a lemon.
    As for eight—eight will get me ten because
I'm hooked on the purity, the plain, old-fashioned
surety of quenching my thirst with the liquids of
weightlessness.

Of course, it's silly to serenade a drink of water with
dumb little ditties, but in a culture dripping with sugar water and
caffeinated rivers, my little poetic streams of consciousness
dribble into tiny tributaries which filleth my cup to the trim.

The Self-centered Shimmy

All silly ditties aside, the free flow of words and ideas onto paper
or into computer fills me with pleasure. Yes, depending upon
my mood, I often word process my problems in a computerized
diary. As lacking in aesthetics as it sounds, I use a disk diary
almost daily. Over the years my keyboard has gone from a
screaming green screen to a lyrical mint julep synthesizer,
becoming as natural to me now as a quill once was to Mary
Shelley. And since I can type a whole lot faster than I can write,
my machine can help me spill out a lot more inky feelings in far
less time.
    Yet, for all my computing and writing, dancing and
water-drinking, in the end it was my inner life that alchemized
and sustained my Thin Lady.
    Erica Jong once said something about good writing
being less inspired by talent than by courage—*the courage to
follow one's creativity into the dark places where it may lead.*

Diary writing takes courage, but truth is a flashlight in the dark cave.

And once I scattered away the dust and cobwebs in my darkest recesses, I could see that I needed to get rid of the bats in my belfry; that is, once I understood my innermost hopes and fears, I needed to reprogram my behavior.

To a great extent, writing works wonders. Yet, if writing provides the flashlight in a dark cave, I could see I needed a pick and shovel to release the gems embedded there in the many layers of the bedrock of my behavior.

I needed a tape recorder.

A lot of my journal entries felt like heart-to-heart talks with myself. Having used other people's meditation tapes to relax and heal, taping my own tête-à-têtes was a natural next step in my liberating dance of self-conscious freedom.

So, I began to redesign myself first on paper, then on tape. After all, I'd already been listening to reel upon reel of internalized, memorized messages from my past. From the loud, rejecting thud of a blacktop street to the bluesy, rap-style jazz I spoke into my mirror. And back to the time a kindergarten teacher teased me that I couldn't "make it" unless I knew a better way to say it, I'd been recording and listening to other, less helpful remembered messages. I was playing back those prerecorded "can'ts" and "shouldn'ts" more often than I was enjoying the sounds of joy!

So, I began to set my diary pep talks to tape. On these recordings, I always spoke to myself in the second person ("you") and gave myself plenty of relaxation cues before making tentative overtures.

Here's an example from one I call "Expand Your Inner Horizon Reduce Your Outer Space":

. . . Now as you continue relaxing, you feel your entire body soften like a pillow. You are your own pillow. Feel the comfort of your being. Snuggle inside yourself; lay your head gently upon the pillow of yourself. Even imagine yourself exhilarated by the childish pillow fights of your playful mind and rest assured that you deserve the best eiderdown feathers for your head and your heart.

In this way my soft and subtle overtures lulled me on to further orchestrate my own change:

. . . And now as you envision a group of circles, feel your own inner power as spheres of influence that have yet to be explored. You draw a circle on your inner paper and begin to feel how good and powerful you really are. Perhaps you let yourself get big in order to feel more important. Perhaps you thought that by taking up a larger space, others would pay more attention to you.

Let yourself draw more concentric circles. These are circles of power. Draw up your goodness, your inherent power, and pour it all onto your inner paper. See your circle of power as a poem, a painting, a ring of good fortune that you can use at any given moment. Know that your inner self is as powerful as those circles. Know that you do not need to be big on the outside to be powerful . . .

And so on.

I made tapes to meet my Fat Lady and to serenade my Thin Woman, to play with my Skinny Kid, and to empower my Super Svelte heroine. And as I listened to those tapes I began to envision a greater diary.

The Interior Shuffle

My inner diary came to me during that drifting state between sleeping and awakening. I like to think of it as a gift from the Guardian of Dreams.

I was lying in bed one morning with two opposing yens —one to get up and write my novel, another to sleep and plot a waking dream or two, that is, to visualize dreamlike pictures, while being awake enough to control the direction of that dream.

I imagined myself walking with great enthusiasm and anticipation down a very long corridor. I saw the entryway as a double-doored dome in a blue, gilded motif.

I decided that my boudoir office lay beyond those doors and as I saw myself pushing open the doors, I continued creating the details of that room. Pillows, windows, murals, even a conga drum appeared in that very special inner space I dubbed Creativity's Cave I imagined it as precisely and as memorably as the room where I was lying awake and dreaming awake.

Here, I had no need of a desk for I had come to this ethereal diary to write slowly, meditatively with a plume and a gold inlaid sketch book. There was a low, glass and painted canvas table made by an artist friend and upon that familiar table I placed a few favorite items from my other office, including a talisman that upon awakening would help to stimulate the memory of this meditation.

Once I had my room decorated to my liking, I saw myself lying down and opening my sketch book. I began turning pages and looking for entries that may have slipped unaware between the covers. Sure enough, scrawled in my worst penmanship was a little note to my subconscious:

"I am not good enough!"

I imagined myself ripping out the page and with little fanfare, tearing it to pieces. Then, with very careful, reflective strokes I wrote:

"I am good enough!"

Unlike the long, wandering, winding roads of my physical diary's real paper pages, my metaphysical diary enjoyed simpler, more direct routes to change.

Now, after years of continuing my visualized journaling, I find my way easily into that inner chamber. From time to time, negative notes pop up as if penned in reverse disappearing ink. But because I own the intimate details of my imagination, I am free to read them and weep, and then destroy those unwanted messages before my psyche can bring them to the forefront and dwell on them.

In my metaphysical diary I create only thoughts I truly choose, with conscious good will toward my life. I read there such entries as very specific prayers, little poems of love and hope, and although I still need to process my daily bread on real paper, my attitude and behavior reflect all the positive inputting in both my diaries.

For if I am what I eat, then surely I am what I write.

The Jerk: Dance of the Human Dodo

Although eccentric was not something I sought to be, nor did I make an attempt to deviate from the norm, I somehow developed a unique style and approach toward life. In retrospect, I believe my variant vision is more a survivor's craft than an artist's design. I am grateful for the freedom eccentricity affords me, even if it sometimes isolates me so that I feel like some kind of an extinct bird.

Because from this, my inherited "dodo's" perch, I have been able to scan my options and locate new paths and clearings in the jungle of my life.

While I was organizing this book into a publishable format, I began to let Thin Linnie stray a bit off course. With a part-time job, a full-time child, and an editorial deadline, I began to neglect exercising, writercising, and preparing the balanced meals that helped me evolve from fat to thin. (I'm sure the irony of a fattening lifestyle accommodating the writing of a book about getting and staying fit would not be lost on the dodo bird!)

But before I lost sight of my intended destination, I began again to write to Thin Linnie:

July 4, 1990

Hey, Thin Linnie,
        Even though I let the Big Baloney sneak back into the front seat, I still feel you at the wheel. But sometimes it feels like you're steering from the back seat, which limits your view of the road ahead and has got to be uncomfortable for you—leaning over the Big Baloney like that.

I guess this auto analogy comes from seeing my reflection in a black shiny car today, knowing that my inner scale registers you slipping over our acceptable weight limit. Still, somehow I saw and felt my reflection as thin.

Fat Lady, Thin Woman. It's all so subjective. Maybe that's a big point of all this. When do I feel thin? More and more I am eliminating pounds from that definition. Thin is a feeling in my stomach. Thin is satisfaction, contentment. Fat feels overstuffed and a bit insatiable. Thin fits my favorite clothes, while fat struggles with the wardrobe of my mind.

I've hung another favorite dress on my door. It is white and wonderful and fringed with shells. It's gotten too tight on the hips to wear. It speaks to me of believing I deserve to be that shapely.

Getting fat accommodates my need to believe in the inner Toni without the outer traps of sorrowful scars or firm muscles. I have accepted my scars and even transformed my feelings about them from pathetic to okay. In the past I have dealt with those scars through a survivor's best defense mechanism— pride. Today on the beach, I felt far less egotistical pride and much more casual acceptance. These last years of journaling have lessened the burden of the cicatrix gnarl.

I believe I can live with my scars and muscles and still feel free enough to fuel my body with healthy food that energizes and nourishes me day by day. I don't need to store fat for the perils of tomorrow.

I believe I can let go my need to control the outcome and let myself be the person who benefits me and my world best.

It is in this sense I believe I deserve the best.

Yes, part of my definition of "the best I can be" is thinness. And part of this Independence Day celebration is claiming my inherent right to eccentricity.

You know, in truth, the dodo bird has been much maligned. The name is colloquially used to describe a person slow to adapt to changing conditions and new ideas; however, historically, the funny-looking bird was a genius of adaptation.

First, the dodo migrated to the isle of Mauritius off the coast of Madagascar, where there were no natural predators. A truly brilliant move! Next, the dodo shortened and thickened his legs and toughened his beak in order to better pursue and devour the abundant insects on the island. And for thousands of years the flightless pigeon thrived.

Of course, in retrospect, giving up his flight plumage and keeping his brilliant tail feathers proved to be the species' undoing as the dodo bird was literally plucked into extinction when humans staked claim to the birds' volcanic fortress.

However, the dodos would have had to have been evolutionary wizards to have outsmarted those human hunters. Human history was moving faster than a dolphin speeding into the web of a tuna net.

But until man came along, the dodo adapted and adapted and survived. Most of all, the dodo dared to be different.

I like thinking of myself as a distant cousin of this extinct, eccentric bird. I aspire to be as different as my true nature desires. And from the sad history of other daring dodos, I have learned how to keep my wings.

I watch for truth in the clouds and write from the wings of my own drama.

I feel those wings attached to strings in the sky and write whatever I want, without worrying whether or not it will "fly."

I imagine loftier viewpoints and write with high hopes.

The dodos may be dead, but the gaudy, gentle inhabitants of Mauritius who germinated the seeds of the Calvaria trees in their excrement and kept the Calvaria alive, inspire those who know the challenge of evolution to spread their wings and change.

The Holistic Hula

I deliberately separated myself upon the pages of my diary; that is, long before I set my story to paper, I severed my ties with society's measuring tape by declining to accept the impossible standards.

Rather than dividing me against myself, though, the Big Baloney, and Thin Linnie, Super Svelte a.k.a. Superjoy, Skinny Kid and Chubby Child, all conspired to make me whole again.

Dissecting my feelings as if they belonged to different people sharing the same skin gave me the distance and perspective I needed to explore those feelings deeply and without censorship.

Imagination thrives on the seemingly unimaginable.

And, it seems my courage expanded when there were more people inside me to brave the dark corners. "The more, the merrier" and "misery loves company" may be clichés, but they are tried and true axioms.

Although I still occasionally write to my various personnas in the second person, these days I mostly write in the first person singular.

July 8, 1990

I have come a long way to get to this plateau of
self-acceptance. I have written a mountain of words
and followed my many streams to the source. I feel
more like an ocean than the scattered islands of
unhappier days.

I enjoy this empathetic view. No "tsks" nor
titters for the circus fat ladies. No envious "ahs" for
the cover girls of Madison Avenue.

I have lost almost a third of my body weight
and gained new characteristics of myself.

Moreover, I know I am more than my body,
even if I am no less than it.

Although my "Diary of a Fat Lady" will never be a
finished book, it is as complete as need be to share it here with
you.

I invite you into my Writercise workshop now, by turning to Part 2, and beginning your own diary, writing to your own
Thin Woman and Fat Lady, and whomever else you may discover under your own cover.

Remember, if I can smile at my scars, and the paralyzed
ballerina can accept her shrunken limbs, and thousands of other
traumatized bodies and souls can look into their own eyes and
find joy and harmony, love and peace, so can you.

Part 2

Writercises:
How to Write Yourself Thin

Hungry Hanna used to hurt
Unless I gave her some dessert
Now Hungry Hanna feels just fine
Knowing she's a pal of mine
A pal who knows cream cheese pie
Is nothing but a big fat lie!

5

Making Contact

Be Kind to Your Fat Lady Friend!

Think of writercising as your inner gym for exercising your emotions and toning up your thoughts. At first, working out with words might be a little difficult. You might even feel like you're sweating it out while getting started or feel a bit awkward the first couple of times. *But hang in there!* Re-creating your body with your mind can become a favorite form of recreation if you relax and invite your muse.

As I mentioned in the introduction, if the thought of writing yourself thin sounds as impossible to you as trying to calculate an astronomical black hole in your weight, then do it à la talkercise. That is, talk the writercises into a tape recorder.

Or if you prefer the visual, do the writercises in your inner diary. (I wake up and fall asleep writing in my subconscious diary. You might want to read Writercise 21, which tells how to create and keep an inner diary.)

Otherwise, if you haven't already bought yourself a big fat notebook, quit reading right now and go get one. A simple spiral will do, but if your style borders on the artistic or if you prefer the freedom of writing without lines, I suggest you treat yourself to a colorful, bound journal or one of those black sketch books from an art supply store. After all, you *are* sketching a new you!

If you do decide upon a fancier model, just make sure the aesthetic look of it doesn't intimidate you. Writing pretty words to match lovely paper is not the main idea here.

As you read further, thoughts will likely come to you that will be good topics for exploring in your diary. So, you'll find spaces to write scattered throughout the following chapters, provided for you to make notes to yourself. Catch a good idea while you can and commit it to paper!

Also, get used to writing in the present tense. You want to change now, not tomorrow. Remember, tomorrow never comes! Think in the here and now and your body will cooperate with the same immediacy.

And remember, this is *your* diary, your solo safari into yourself. No one else is invited to be present at your banquet, not even your mother. You know, the woman with the trick mirror, the one who takes 10 pounds off your image whenever she invites you to the family feast.

And if you are concerned about someone else reading your private, intimate thoughts, by all means hide or lock up your diary.

Remember, as you take your turn filling in your own blanks, bridging—and closing—the gap between your fat and thin selves, let the way you write be as natural as the way you speak. Don't strain for ideas or worry about grammar or spelling. Let whatever flows into your mind drip down to your pen and spill out onto the paper. The best way to rid yourself of self-censorship is to write fast, without stopping to read what you've written. The words don't need to make sense to anyone but you.

There is no right or wrong diary entry.

Writing to your Fat Lady and Thin Woman can be a wonderful and sometimes painful journey into real and imagined rejection. Yet, only by facing all the bugaboos in your inner closet will it ever become a safe place for all your separate selves.

Besides the writercises in this book, I also invite you to write down all your random fat feelings. Morning, noon, and in lieu of a midnight snack. Before and after meals or whenever you can get a moment, scribble a few lines.

If you tend to snack from boredom or loneliness, keep your diary in a kitchen drawer. Write your own encouraging words to help your Fat Lady the next time she wanders near the fridge. Tell yourself the truth about why you are there in the kitchen. Sometimes just a few sentences make the difference between whether you eat a loaf or a slice of bread.

If you live alone or with understanding housemates, print a mantra (statement) from your Fat Lady and tack it to a wall. Keep it simple so you can repeat it silently throughout your day.

Some of my favorite mantras from my Writercise groups are:

- Twenty years ago, I could have modeled for Botticelli.
- Beauty and the obese! That's me!
- I have a right to be fat. So there!

Whenever you pick up your pen, think to yourself, "I am willing to meet myself and change"—change meaning either in body shape or personal self-image or both. Accepting and loving your present self can be the first step in the process of change or, if you choose, the end result—certainly a result worth celebrating. You may decide you like yourself just the way you are. Self-acceptance is a change for the better and as rewarding as any weight loss.

Either way, the more you write, the more you will discover. Discovery leads to change and change is your aim or you wouldn't have bought this book.

Don't be afraid to be frank about your problems. I found that asking questions in the diary sometimes left me with wide open blanks. If the answers did not pop up immediately, they often would slip into place while I was vacuuming or lazing in a bath.

If you like to play with words, have fun doing so, but don't get so carried away that upon rereading you won't understand your images.

If you begin writing off onto a tangent all your own, track it wherever it leads. Do not feel coerced to follow any of the writercises to the letter. The instructions are intended to head you in the right direction, but you are your own best navigator.

Always give yourself a comfortable writing space where you are not likely to be disturbed. Since I wrote lying down during much of my adolescence as well as my convalescence, I particularly enjoy writing in bed.

In truth, successful journaling is whatever works for you.

There's only one hard and fast rule to follow when making contact with your Fat Lady: BE KIND!

Writercise 1:
You've Got a Friend

Get off to a comfortable writing nook. Before beginning, inhale deeply. Let yourself believe that you've got a friend. A friend who wants what's best for you. A friend who believes that being overweight is what's best for you. And up until now, it *has* been what's right for you or you wouldn't be thus.

However, you are now ready to reexamine your needs. Together you and your Fat Lady can choose whether to continue being fat on the outside. Together you will decide how to rewrite yourself. How to reshape your body. How to plot a happier ending.

Take a few deep breaths, confident that you can discover in the pages of your Fat Lady journal the mystery of who you are, who you want to be, who you can be. Picture yourself extending an understanding hand, a loving mind to your Fat Lady. She takes it because you are her friend.

Over the next five days you are to write a series of letters to your Fat Lady. Begin each time by rereading the beginning of this writercise.

LETTER 1:

Give your Fat Lady a special name. Tell her something you like about her.

Ask her who she is and wait for a reply. Be ready to write the first thoughts that come to mind. Ask her how she feels about her body. Be patient if she is slow to respond and don't reject anything that comes to mind. Write it without censoring her (your) words.

Ask about her fears. Ask her what is frightening about losing weight. Address each and every issue she raises with gentle reassurance and love.

End with a word of hope. (Please avoid making stressful promises which often lead to disappointment.) Thank your Fat Lady for sharing with you and remember, you've got a friend.

When you finish, wrap your arms around yourself and give your Fat Lady a wonderful hug. (Do this or some version of it, after each letter.)

LETTER 2:

Greet your Fat Lady like an old friend.

Ask her to describe any stress going on in her life. Try to offer constructive solutions.

Ask her to list what she ate today and how each selection left her feeling. If she expresses self-loathing, forgive her. Ask her to help you figure out less harmful substitutes.

Write out a perfect day of meals that would satisfy both your Fat Lady's appetite and your self-esteem. Choose a day on which you could conceivably enjoy that perfect food-fare. Ask your Fat Lady to adopt this as a once-a-week menu.

Thank your Fat Lady for sharing herself with you.

LETTER 3:

(Before beginning, tear letter 1 from your diary, put it in an envelope and, without rereading it, mail it to yourself.)

Now, pick up your pen and give your Fat Lady a heartfelt welcome.

Create the perfect fantasy day for your Fat Lady. What would she do if there were no mention of food in it? Of course, she will eat; however, eating is so immaterial to her perfect day, she need not think about it nor mention it.

Describe that day, in the now and in detail, as if it were actually happening.

Stop a moment and read over your fantasy. Is there a way you could make some or all of this perfect day happen? Choose a day within the next week and write out the date, suggesting that date for putting your perfect day into action.

Sign off cordially.

LETTER 4:

(Mail letter 2 to yourself.)

Begin by greeting your Fat Lady. "Hello and how do you do?"

For many diarists, this next letter is the toughest. Do it anyway. A pen pal can lay all her cards on the table and trust the process to sort them and deal back a fair hand.

Write out a history of your Fat Lady's ups and downs. How did your Fat Lady feel each time she got fat after being thin? What events, if any, occurred simultaneously? What was the reaction from people around her and how did that make her feel?

Tell her you understand—and then really try to.

Ask your Fat Lady to visit you often in the pages of your diary.

LETTER 5:

(Mail letter 3.)

After your salutation, talk about physical exercise. Ask your Fat Lady how she feels about walking, bicycling, swimming. Does she prefer indoor or outdoor activity? Have there been any past problems regarding exercise that she needs to share?

Ask her to choose some form of fitness she can do for fifteen minutes a day, something aerobic enough to get the heart rate up and raise your metabolism, which helps your body burn more calories throughout the entire day, even while sleeping. (A simple means of figuring metabolic heart rate for your age group is detailed in Covert Bailey's book *Fit or Fat*. Also, remember that it's always a good idea to consult your physician before beginning any exercise program.)

Imagine how she will feel after a month of walking (or biking). Write out her reaction.

Thank her for creating this active scenario for you. Sign off and stretch like a cat, enjoying your perfectly purring body.

Finish mailing your letters, one each day. If you wish, continue writing letters and mailing them to yourself as the need arises. When you receive your letters, read and reread them. Again, make no promises, but be open to the suggestions from your special friend. As problems arise in the diary, you can make lists of possible solutions.

For example, Suzanne feared that if she became thin, her best friend Teri would be intimidated. Suzanne felt dependent on Teri's friendship. Suzanne was asked to make a list of possible solutions, even those she might not be inclined to follow at the moment. Suzanne's list included:

1. Explain to Teri why I want to lose weight. Tell her I'm afraid of losing her friendship if I get thinner. Ask her if it would matter.
2. If it doesn't matter—GREAT. If it does, quit losing weight.

3. Make new friends, ones who will accept me and all my changes.
4. Help Teri start her own Fat Lady diary.

Even though Suzanne said that either dumping her diet or her best friend were out of the question, she felt comforted to know she did, in fact, have some options. In the end, Suzanne made so many significant lifestyle changes that Teri felt estranged from Suzanne and began avoiding her. However, by that time Suzanne's life was full enough to absorb the loss.

When writing, keep in mind the emphasis upon empathy. In the Writercise workshops, sometimes women have balked at approaching the fat part of themselves with empathy and kindness, assuming they would never decide to diet if they accepted their Fat Lady. Yet, befriending the Fat Lady is the only way I know to enlist full cooperation from the self.

Besides, do you really want to hate any part of yourself?

That first initial contact with your Fat Lady may at first prove hostile. Yet, just as exposure and understanding worked to lessen the cold war between embittered nations, so will writing with an open heart and mind bring about a truly lasting peace for you and your Fat Lady.

Marla had been my creative writing teacher and we had kept in touch over the years. When I told her how journal writing had helped me shape up and stabilize my weight, she encouraged me to teach my process to others.

Marla, herself an avid diarist, originally came to my workshops to lend me moral support. She thought she had all her fat issues covered until she got there.

Even with all her lines and letters, Marla had never attempted to make contact with that Fat Lady within. And as Marla learned, sometimes that Fat Lady has been sitting on her heels, just waiting for you to try to reach her with words of hope.

Here is part of Marla's letter:

Dear Fat Lady,

You feel far away and separate from me. I cannot accept you because everything I have been told for forty-plus years makes you unacceptable to be—to me, I mean. I wrote *to be* by accident—or was it? Somehow at my core it always seems to come back to my right *to be*. Maybe because Mother made no secret that I was a "little mistake" and that her unplanned pregnancy at forty caused considerable unhappiness in the family, even if, once I was born, I became the "little princess."

Fat Lady, you really had a hard time—*have* a hard time accepting and loving yourself. Toni's meditation was so lovely. She tried to show you that I, your Fat Lady, have a right *to be* and am a beautiful part of you. You can't seem to get healed from your feelings of being an unwanted child. I want you to listen to Toni's meditation over and over—maybe even make your own tape. You need to work on self-acceptance—to learn to love yourself—to heal that mother wound within. You need to learn to love and embrace yourself. As you work on your nurturing issues, you won't have to feed yourself to show you love yourself.

I'd really like to love you. I wish I could have given you a big hug during the meditation as Toni advised. Lord knows, you need a hug. You need to be told you are okay. If your husband can love you when you're 50 pounds overweight, why can't you love yourself?

Why not indeed? As Marla learned, she had mother-rooted insecurities that translated into obsessions with food. Marla used the diary to give birth to another self, one with the right *to be.*

Mother roots run deep and may take a lifetime to retrain.

Consider another type of mother-rooted dinner bell that women from a different background hear. Diana came to Writercise 30 pounds overweight and angry at her spreading stomach and oversized waist. In spite of my instructions, she regularly scolded her Fat Lady. Her Fat Lady was so busy defending herself that Diana learned little about the midnight food forays adding to her bulk. At the group's urging, Diana finally wrote an apology and a week later, this emerged:

Late at night, the Fat Lady croaks through my dreams.
I hear her. "Ribbet, ribbet, ribbet," I hear her webbed
feet slapping tiles, jumping down the aisles of a
supermarket. She looks for tadpoles. Sweet and sour
tadpoles. Tadpoles in a can. Fresh and frozen,
freeze-dried and instant and TV tadpole dinners. I
open a zip-lock bag of tadpole chips, but instead find
the Fat Lady. She croaks up at me with bullfrog eyes.
    "Where are my tadpoles?" she asks. "Where
are my tadpoles?"

When Diana shared this with the class, I wasn't convinced that Diana had broken her Fat Lady's wall of silence until she explained.

"Those tadpoles are the babies I will never have!"

Diana had had a hysterectomy at an early age and had never mourned the loss. As a matter of fact, she forgot she had ever wanted children. Fifteen years later Diana looked like a pregnant eggplant.

What the mind tries to hide, the body will often confirm.

Your body is the statue sculpted by your mind.

Now Diana has nicknamed her Fat Lady "Big Mama" and writes to her often. She says it may take another notebook to grieve over the babies she will never have, but now she rarely tries to stuff her maternal feelings with food.

Diana's Fat Lady was actually mothering and nurturing her long-forgotten pregnant longings. Diana's Fat Lady was being a very good friend.

Diana also quit berating her stomach for getting fat. Besides providing the illusion of pregnancy, her bloated belly was also trying to save her from a possible famine. After all, the stomach is a primitive organ. Diana's nightly gorging cued her body to save up for lean times. Like her ancestors, Diana could survive if she had plenty of fat in reserve.

Diana wrote:

Dear Stomach,

You have expanded to accommodate my desire to have babies. Thank you for trying to fulfill my dreams but I can't become pregnant. And food fat is not baby fat.

So you can quit trying to fool me. I'm working on my feelings of loss. I'll be okay.

You know, I have hated you for being fat and loved you for looking pregnant. How unfair. You were storing fat for me and my fantasy and perhaps even, stashing life-sustaining fat in case of famine. But listen, Stomach, I'm in no danger of starving.

Your body has its favorite storage shelves. Wherever this is for you, the overstocked pantry is the first place you gain weight and the last place you lose it. It is often the part of your body you resent the most.

Directing hostile resentment at any part of your body only causes anxiety. Dr. Nancy Bryan writes in her wonderfully enlightening book, *Thin Is a State of Mind*, "If we boiled down all the internal obstacles to losing weight into one word, that word would be 'anxiety.' "

I couldn't agree more.

Anger is anxiety wearing a mask of snarls. Many people try to stuff their self-directed anger. Food, however, is just a bandage, a mummy's wrapper that binds up the real hurt.

Fortunately, your diary is a safe haven for facing your resentments and unrealistic body fantasies. Keep in mind, however, that you may slim down but you won't grow any taller.

Let go those leggy delusions. Just as I found release in writing to my scars, Diana set her stomach free and so did Lane who discovered she hated her "big bad belly," but not because it looked like she'd swallowed a watermelon. Lane thought it was that simple until she began writing to her stomach and realized what she hated was the stomach cancer that had killed her mother.

Lane ate constantly hoping to keep her stomach so stuffed there wouldn't be any room for cancerous cells to grow. The diary helped her release the sorrow of losing her mother as well as much of her own fear of the disease.

The rational mind can sort the mess of misconceptions that our emotions often tangle. Diary writing allows you to see the tangle in its proper perspective and then to reshape the changeable and accept the unchangeable.

Notes

Writercise 2:
Let Me Hear Your Body Talk

Sit quietly a moment and get in touch with your body. Briefly close your eyes and listen to your breath fill your lungs. Listen as your body relaxes.

Is one or more of your body parts aching to speak out?

Open your eyes and begin writing to that specific body part.

If you are unhappy about the way a particular part of your body stores fat, talk to your disappointment. Let it talk back. If you are angry, express that anger. Write from those feelings, and yet be willing to acknowledge that your body is not the enemy. Your body is doing the best it can.

Set your anger free.

If you are addressing a particularly oversized part of yourself, talk realistically about your expectations. Tell it how you would like to reshape it.

Ask it if there is a reason it cannot slim into your ideal expectations and listen for a reply. Be honest about what you hear. If your expectations are not reasonable, write why they are not.

Now think of something good, a compliment to pay that body part, something sincere and encouraging. After all, your out-of-shape legs still get you from point A to point B.

Write to that body part as often as you need, especially if you find yourself hating the way it looks. Write until you learn to love it simply for being a part of you.

Think of Theresa, who wrote that even though her upper arms were as fat as thighs, she and her sister had a lot of laughs pretending her flabby arm was a guitar. Julia would play the strings of Theresa's guitar to the delight of their children.

Filter your body language through your understanding heart.

Remember that magazine experiment I mentioned earlier where women estimated the size of their hips by spreading their hands as wide as they imagined their girth to be? Almost without exception, women saw their hips as considerably larger than they actually were.

Perhaps you are misjudging your hips or thighs or arms.

Tune into the way you feel about your body and you'll be ready to interpret the murmurs of more than just your hungry stomach.

Perhaps you'll hear your mind fine-tuning your body with forgiveness and gratitude.

From the notebooks of Laura del Fuego:

Ode to my Hips

Mounds of flesh
prodigious protrusions
deliciously adipose
cellulite lumps
smooth as oysters
fatty tissue that
carries boxes babies
and small bags of fruit
and sways to the music of future dreams

Hope
hula dancing in Hawaii
or was it an Arabian night
a belly or two
too big too soft
too yielding
they say jelly and jam
begin that way
satin smooth
pudding
papayas pineapples
promises promises promises
like rolling hills
spreading out into
the lush green spring
of purple skies
nutmeg cinnamon clove
sage and curry
ripe scented lemon
growing and shifting
into time elements
this life-giving fat

Notes

Writercise 3:
See Yourself Thin

It should be about time to meet your Thin Woman.

That's right—Thin Linnie, Skinny Minnie, Slim Kim, Boney Maroni—whatever you opt to call your slender side, you do possess a svelte silhouette.

"But I've always been fat!" you object?

Okay. I was a skinny kid until pink pleats came along. Still I felt fat. If you once believed there was a Chubby Child trapped inside a Skinny Kid, why couldn't there just as well be a slinkier you prowling your mental corridors? (Why not indeed? That's what your diary is helping you discover.)

Consider the dichotomous nature of our minds. Haven't you ever had an ugly moment right in the middle of a pretty day? Or felt like Einstein one minute and the village idiot the next?

A Fat Lady and Thin Woman living in the same body isn't that far-fetched. It's actually just a slight stretch of the imagination.

Right now, close your eyes a moment and let your Thin Woman take shape.

Visualizing your inner Thin Woman is only one part imagination. The rest is sheer stubborn determination. Write about your Thin Woman. Think about her. Talk about her. Pretend she's looking back at you when you look in the mirror. Talk to that reflection. The more substance you give your thin character, the more readily she will walk off the pages of your diary and inherit your body. One day you'll hear her whisper, "I'd rather have an orange." You'll be surprised to find yourself reaching for fruit instead of cake, just like I did.

Many women lose lots of weight and still feel fat. Often they gain the weight back in order to fill out this inner vision of themselves. If you already feel and think thin before you are physically thin, you'll be able to move through life as a truly thin person when you reach your weight goal.

Maxwell Maltz, author of the classic book on visualization, *Psycho-Cybernetics*, says that "experimental and clinical psychologists have proved beyond a shadow of a doubt that the human nervous system cannot tell the difference between an 'actual' experience and an experience imagined vividly and *in detail*."

Or to put it another way—what you see is what you get!

See yourself thin and healthy and your behavior and body will comply with your vision.

Janet had problems pretending, let alone imagining a Thin Woman. As a chubby child and obese adolescent, she had no reference for a thinner self.

Her usually long sentences simply came to a halt whenever she tried to personify her Thin Woman:

> I am a normal weight. I'm healthy and look better. My thighs don't embarrass me. My stomach doesn't pop out. Even when I visit Mother I don't take seconds. I am no longer intimidated by grocery store clerks. I don't care what they think of the food I choose. I'm not fat.

In more than a dozen entries, Janet never referred to herself as thin, even though I had stressed that thin is a relative term to be defined by the perception in each individual's mind. Neither did she voluntarily write to her Thin Woman except in specific writercises.

She did, however, write volumes to her Fat Lady. The breakthrough came when her Fat Lady started talking about her Thin Woman:

I am Fat Jan and I am afraid to let go of this weight. I hold on to it like I do my children and my husband, afraid the world might swallow them up.

If Thin Jan were here, I am afraid she too would be swallowed up by a busy world. Fat, I stay home and give to my family. Thin I may begin to join clubs and shop for beautiful clothes. Thin, I might be too selfish to give to the kids. I am afraid that Thin Jan would be empty of her maternal tendencies. Like my mother who was always too busy working to care whether I was fat or thin.

Oh boy, does this ever sound like spilt milk. I am not my mother. I should be able to trust the love I have for my family. Maybe some things will change. Who knows, maybe I would go get a part-time job outside the house. After all I am not my mother.

Whether as Fat Jan or Thin Jan, I love my family. I need to love myself enough to trust that love and give myself some choices.

Janet says that this entry launched her on a roller coaster ride, one she'd been avoiding a long, long time. For Janet, her issue was simple and she spent the rest of the six-week workshop (and hopefully following months) working out her "bad mother blues."

Let's begin to prepare a space for your Thin Woman to emerge. Design (and later write a description of) the environment that most suits the Thin Woman you would like to be. I recommend a space where your Thin Woman can be active, because exercise aids and abets your thin dreams. Also, you are not a still-life snapshot but an active, moving organism. See yourself living a drama, not posing like a cardboard cut-out of yourself.

Close your eyes and imagine yourself thin. What do you look like? See your face as it is, only thinner. Even if the visual image you have is fleeting, give it life by believing in it. (Easy for you to say, you retort? Maybe so, but you can make a beginning by mouthing the words, even if they are only spoken in the privacy of your consciousness. Don't believe me? Give it a try, because the process does work.) Over the next few weeks, for a few seconds, dozens of times each day, imagine yourself thin like this.

Now, lace your thin fingers around your pen and begin writing. Start by giving your Thin Woman a name, keeping in mind, of course, that she is still you. Describe her. How does she wear her hair? What kind of clothes does she wear?

Plan a day for your Thin Woman. Remember to write in the now, the present tense. Begin with waking in the morning. How does it feel to stretch your lithe, lean body?

What do you have for breakfast? Think nutritiously thin.

Do you go to work at the same job as you do now? (If not, you need to review your career goals sometime soon.)

Do you walk briskly or bicycle for enjoyment?

Describe what you pack for lunch.

Go shopping for clothes. How does it feel to try on new fashions? How do other people react? If their reactions stir discomfort within you, write about your reaction to theirs.

If you are afraid of your thin body, explore your fear with words.

Sharon had trouble visualizing her thinner self. After questioning, it became apparent that she was trying to consciously force a picture of her desired self, instead of relaxing and letting her inner mind provide the image.

Sharon didn't need to direct her vision. Before she ever closed her eyes, her inner self knew what she was seeking—a clear image of her Thin Woman. She needed to learn how to meditate, because meditation is letting go.

Meditation is like going to the theater. Your conscious mind selects the movie, yet you don't know exactly what's going to happen. You need only to kick back, relax, and view the pictures on your subconscious reel.

The good news is Sharon began deep breathing and quit straining. Within weeks, she was able to write about the image of her thinner self, as she walked briskly through her inner landscape:

> Seeing myself thin like this absolutely convinces me that there really is a Skinny Minnie inside my Fat Cat, trying to get out. I've been walking a lot again. The vision inspires me to walk more, and the walking sketches in more details of Skinny Minnie's portrait. And I don't need to lock myself away to meditation either. Walking is meditation. Cooking supper, driving to work, washing the dishes—it's all meditation when I relax and let something quiet and still inside come out.

Unlike Sharon, Marla easily visualized her Thin Woman. However, seeing isn't always believing . . .

> I want to believe in you, Thin Woman. I really do! During the meditation, I really felt thin, serene, and lovely. As for the fear part, I realized the major thing holding me back is that I feel thin people have to be constantly "on guard." They don't get to indulge themselves without carefully measuring the price and fasting later. I'm pretty convinced I could not stay thin

without constant effort and a complete loss of the pleasures of food.

But is this true?

It took me more than a year to gain back the weight after that crash diet, so I wonder if I would be able to solve the emotional needs to overeat and learn how to better deal with my emotions and simply never eat ONE bite more than I really want or need. Is there a chance this would work?

And just a few days after writing this, Marla found some guidance in another entry:

I am feeling really different about my "problems." I am completely turned around in my thinking, so that losing weight no longer seems a hopeless task, nor am I frightened by the prospect of discipline and hunger. A very significant change seemed to come about with my search for the "skinny kid." The tape I made for myself, my understanding of what sweets really meant to me, and my decision to simply "turn off" that connection have made what feels like a major change of attitude. I feel confident and optimistic.

You see, you cannot conscript your subconscious mind to serve your conscious desires. But, if you extend a loving invitation, your inner self will volunteer for duty. If that sounds hard to believe, I extend to you a loving invitation to try it. I think you'll actually be amazed at the depth of the change in your feelings.

Notes

Writercise 4:
Oh, You Must Have Been a Beautiful Doll!

Let's really cut some fat out now!

Get out the kids' crayons, the old, colored pencils, some markers, or simply find a lead pencil or pen. Get a large sheet of paper and lay it out in front of you. Now close your eyes and picture your Fat Lady. What does she look like? What kind of expression is on her face? What does she have in her hand? Keep your eyes closed long enough to notice what it is she is carrying.

Open your eyes and begin drawing your Fat Lady. Remember, she's your friend and you don't need to worry about offending her. Also, don't worry about the artistic accuracy. Just have fun with it. Draw round circles if that's all you can manage, and don't forget to draw that item she had in hand.

Now color or shade her. Add some life to her cheeks and flair to her clothes.

When you are through, take out your diary and write to your Fat Lady. Is there anything in particular you need to tell her? Explain what it is she holds in her hand. Why does she need it or want it? Are you glad she brought it? Would you like to change it into something else?

Now take a few moments to close your eyes and imagine your Thin Woman. How does she look? What one item does she carry?

When you have a clear impression of her, take your pencil and begin outlining your Thin Woman inside the contours of your Fat Lady. Does she carry the same thing in her hand or do you need to change it?

When you finish defining your Thin Woman, take a pair of scissors and trim off a little bit of your Fat Lady so that she becomes more like your Thin Woman. As you cut, tell yourself what you are trying to remove with those scissors besides fat.

Over the next few weeks or months, return to your paper doll whenever you feel the need to rid yourself of some emotional weight.

Every time you cut away a bit more, turn to your diary and write about it. What does the loss feel like? If you are losing weight as well, explore any feeling of deprivation or sacrifice you might be feeling.

If you are like most women, you are a complicated set of contradictions. You might be glad for the weight you are losing while resenting what that weight represents.

You lose weight, your favorite clothes no longer fit.

You lose weight, your heavier friends avoid you; your husband acts jealous; your secure morals are challenged.

A recurring theme in Janet's diary was the fights her mother and she had over her weight. Two years ago Janet had gone on a vigorous diet, getting down to her ideal weight. As the weight dropped off, so did the confrontations. You would think that subdued relations with her mother would be the pot of gold at the end of her diet. Janet thought so too. However, when the familiar interaction with her mother ceased, nothing came along to replace it.

She puzzled on the pages of her diary:

My mother's visits became awkward and strained. It's like she had nothing to say to me anymore. She used to bring me diet books and quote success stories from newspaper ads. Then she'd begin criticizing. Everything I ate was all wrong for me. Why didn't I join a health spa or jog like the girl next door. When I got down to my Svelte Yvette, I didn't miss the fights but I hated the silence between us.

Sometimes the familiar, even the uncomfortably familiar, is less threatening than the unknown. Like the "bad child" who believes that even negative attention is better than no attention, Janet gained back her weight.

After trimming her paper doll, Janet wrote the following:

> As I cut away my Large Marge, I cut away my anger.
> I am angry at Mother. In all those baby pictures I
> looked like a stuffed pig. Mother was forever
> compensating for the fact that Father deserted us.
> Maybe that's the truth about our relationship. It's not
> the weight I can't let go, it's my anger. And Mother's
> silence is her own guilt. I do not own it.
>
> I like succeeding. I hate myself for letting
> Mother manipulate me. I am Svelte Yvette and if
> Mother never talks to me again, I will learn to accept
> the silence between us.

Losing weight means just that—losing. Figure out what else you might be losing in those inches and pounds and you might just find a way to win through losing.

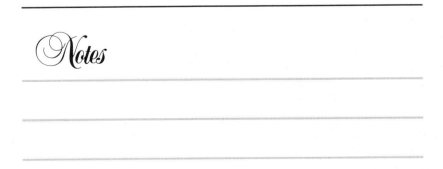

Notes

Notes

Writercise 5:
Pen Out

Win through losing! What a Zen-ful idea. To win because you allow yourself to lose. To lose, to let go, and yet to feel like a winner instead of a loser, because fat is more than the accumulation of stockpiled energy. Fat is a storehouse for emotions, emotion that when expressed can take the fat along with it.

Worst among these is anger. Anger left to brood breeds fat. A few years back I worked briefly as a diet counselor, weighing, charting, and counseling dieters and doing so daily. After a few months I began to notice that literally everyone who reported experiencing stress, especially when they reacted with anger, experienced no weight loss and occasionally even slight gains, regardless of how closely they adhered to the diet plan.

One dieter who began keeping a diary noted that same pattern prevalent in her own progress and began to write letters and dialogues expressing her anger whenever a frustrating incident occurred so that anger never had an opportunity to fester.

For example, Pam wrote the following shortly after an argument with a boyfriend:

September 5, 1987

We rarely go anywhere unless I make the plans. It feels like he doesn't care enough to pick up a newspaper or a phone, invest some energy in us. From dinner reservations to inviting over friends, our social life is in my lap. I'm angry at him but I really should be angry with myself for playing social director and for allowing him to simply drop by planless and penniless. So, he's saving money for a down payment on a house! He could pack a picnic and scout a new hiking path for us to share.

　　And what do I do about it? I nag. I nag and nag and in the end allow him to drop by without any plan of action.

Although Pam never successfully changed that part of her relationship, Pam said the journal provided an outlet for anger that would otherwise have sent her scurrying for sugar.

　　In a similar situation, Marla recalled the night her mother sent home a friend of Marla's, cancelling a promised sleep-over because Marla would not eat her vegetables. She wrote:

I am so angry! I hate you—I hate you—I hate you! It's not my fault. You just can't be this angry over my not eating canned peas! You're making me sick. You make my head hurt. It's wrong of you to insist on controlling me this way! I'm not your little baby anymore and I don't care how darling and perfect I was when you could dress me and feed me . . .

　　The Fat Lady seems to understand how and when your pain began. It was very painful when you recalled that night when your parents punished you by making your friend go home. Reliving the memory allowed me to feel again and somehow rethink the experience.

Marla feels that writing out old anger released some of the sting. It also let her comfort herself in the way she wanted her mother to.

Try to write out anger and annoyance before these have a chance to stimulate your appetite, for anger surely is one of the guiltiest of saboteurs.

Gisela has been angry for a very long time. For her it began when as a young girl she grew taller than all the boys in her class. They taunted her for being tall and fat, even though she was more a big girl than actually fat.

Gisela wrote pages of biting prose that helped her let go the anger she felt toward those little boys and later the men who one way or another seemed to say that she wasn't thin or pretty enough.

Gisela's mantra was "I have a right to be fat. So there!" Later she wrote:

> I'm eating out of rebellion. Yet when I rebel against something, I'm still as run by whatever it is I'm rebelling against. It's almost like by rebelling against something, I'm giving it power over me. I guess the best thing to do when something riles me is to just go my own way without rebelling or accepting. Just be me . . .

Growing up large, Gisela has had more than her share of guilt. Her diary is teaching her to let herself eat and enjoy food without guilt.

Gisela's entry after a late-night snack with friends demonstrates how writing can defuse the bomb that so many of us build into our everyday eating. Gisela wrote:

> Last night I ate some stuff that I shouldn't have. I went with three friends to an art show and afterwards

we stopped at a restaurant and stuffed ourselves. The other three ladies all ordered dinners. I love Mexican food and even though I was not hungry I ordered chips and dip. Really I'd wanted a big gooey cheesy dish. Still, I ate too much and even took home a doggy bag full of leftovers. I really felt awful to eat so much but I guess I should pat myself on the back for not eating more. After all, I could have ordered a combination plate *and* chips and dip.

Whether you work at home or in an office, self-directed anger earns high ratings as a CEO (Calorie Eat Out).

And there's no need to eat yourself to the top when you can write your own memos and pass the anger to your paper.

Remember back to a time when you stuffed yourself silly. Try to remember what you ate. Remember how you felt afterwards. Relive that totally, unbelievably, stuffed-pig feeling. Get in touch with the rage, the indignation, and disbelief, the irate self-hate.

I know, I know, good little girls don't get angry and never, ever hate, at least not so that others can see. Well, this is between you, me, and a piece of paper, and if you don't let it out somehow, you're going to have to stuff it down with something —something heavy enough to anchor all that anger like some chunky piece of chocolate.

So, go ahead, gnash your teeth, get miffed, huff and puff and bark at the moon! Call your Fat Lady names. That's right— get downright nasty. Unload your hostility, shove it down the shaft of your pen! Or let it flow like notes through a flute . . . Whatever your style, just let your anger out.

And as you write, try to be in touch with the part of your body that stores anger. Whether it be the hollow pit of your stomach or the tense knots of your shoulder blades, feel anger loosen its hold on your body as you release it, rather than stuffing food in on top of it.

Don't end your writing on a negative note, though. Always remember to forgive your Fat Lady and apologize for any abuses you may have heaped on her.

Rewrite that anger. Turn it into something else.

Next time, and anytime thereafter, that you feel anger poisoning something inside you, tighten your stomach—not into an angry clinch but with energizing, rejuvenating strength. Imagine your anger as your fat. Now, let it dissolve into sweat as you exercise the muscles of your mind.

And anytime you find yourself in the throes of an all-out pig-out, remember you can stop eating whenever you choose and pen out instead.

Notes

Notes

Writercise 6:
Fat Lady Fit

Here's where your Fat Lady gets even. Now it's her turn to rail and rage against this thinner, slimmer beauty pageant of weights and measurements. Now is the time to blast those magazines with models so thin their hip bones could slice the chocolate cake on the next page. This is where your Fat Lady gets a chance to rake over the coals all those easier, faster, fattier foods, and metabolism so slow it could lose a race to a bottle of ketchup.

Or as Patty put it:

> . . . My roommate eats like a cow or a cowboy after a roundup. If that were me I'd have to lock myself in a sweat box for three days. All she has to do to keep shamelessly skinny is to constantly kick one leg as she sits there and somehow that soups up her metabolism. It's not fair . . .

Amanda had other fumes to vent:

> . . . All those lousy magazines with their boy-shaped models telling me I was a fat teen-ager! I wasn't fat. Now I'm fat. I spent my high school years hating my size eleven body because New York wouldn't feature anyone larger than a size seven. Now what I wouldn't give to fit in a size eleven. I really hate what the media does to women!

Ellen found her husband in her direct line of fire:

Last night the jerk insisted on going to Hot Chile's.
He knows there's nothing innocent on their menu and
that I can never resist their avocado dip and chips. He
hates my thighs and knows I'm trying so hard, but his
belly comes first! He sits around the house spooning
ice cream into his smug little mouth without caring
that minted chocolate chip is my favorite flavor. He's
so thoughtless!

And Gisela dumped her share of rage against the injustice of a male-oriented society:

. . . I sometimes have trouble seeing men as human
beings. I hear about them beating up their wives and
abusing their children. I know these are reverse
chauvinistic reactions, but it just seems that too many
men do horrible things. They molest children and
build Star Wars to destroy everything. They
discriminate against women in the work place, build
up drug empires, and nerve gas. They pollute the
environment and cut down forests. They have all the
political and social power . . .

And so on, until Gisela came around to understanding
that "men are just as weak and frail as we are." Forgiveness for
the young boys who taunted her eventually came for Gisela
through her love for her young son.

Anger left to stew can thicken your pot. Once expressed, especially on the pages of a diary that cannot strike back or take offense, anger becomes a watered-down cup of bitters, yet a cup of bitters that no longer steeps in your head and stimulates your appetite.

Make a list of things about being fat in a thin world and about getting and staying thin that infuriates your Fat Lady. Consider these possibilities:

> magazine models and television cuties
> skinny friends who always order dessert
> husbands who criticize your thighs
> lovers who criticize your low-cal cooking
> people who stare
> people who pretend you're not there

As you write away your anger, continue concentrating on tightening a part of your body that needs a calisthenic boost. Then, next time your skinny friend orders a piece of pecan pie, instead of drooling in envy and anger, tighten up your thighs, and remember what your hostility really means and how you've redefined it.

Now that you're rewriting your feelings, feel free to reshape your body.

Notes

Notes

6

Making Friends

Look, Ma! No Blame!

Do you have reason to believe that someone else started your butterball rolling? Someone who may have meant to nourish but instead overfed you?

Parents who lifted the spoon to your mouth during those first few helpless, baby years actually contributed to the accumulation (or lack) of future fat cells. Scientists now claim that an adult's capacity to gain weight positively correlates to the fat they built up as infants and children.

Like a balloon, those fat cells may have enlarged and shrunk half a dozen times during your lifetime and just like that overblown balloon, those cells get easier to inflate each time you lose and gain weight. Once inflated, even a long skinny balloon refills with less and less effort—which is why some people lose 10 pounds only to gain back 15. Fat cells stand ready with open mouths and stretched stomachs.

As unfair as it may seem, we are all stuck (and/or blessed) with the body our parents designed for us, first by their genetic heritage and later by their dietetic regimen.

That's enough to make any Fat Lady bite the hand that once fed her! And yet, instead of facing that primal point of blame (and thus finding a way to let it go), many of us stuff it down with all the familiar foods we were stuffed with as children, and then some.

Take Harriet, for instance. Harriet's mother was constantly praising her young grandson for cleaning his plate, sometimes even applauding wildly, "as if he'd just played 'Hot Cross Buns' on the piano instead of merely eating them!"

Harriet had been an overindulged and overfed youngster who went from a chubby adolescent to a young woman who dieted, lost, and regained close to 200 pounds in fifteen years. Her relationship with her mother had been strained ever since the night of her senior prom when Harriet's dress tore along the back seam and her mother made a comment about Harriet's appetite for food being stronger than her desire to be attractive.

Criticism became more frequent as Harriet moved out on her own and later began her own family. Harriet assumed that by ignoring her mother's derision, she was untouched by it. However, as she began to write about the way her mother fussed over her son's performance at the dinner table, her anger grew stronger and more defined.

Finally, Harriet wrote:

I'd forgotten so many of the awful things Mother said to me about being fat. I guess I thought I deserved them. After all, I did get fatter right before the prom. Toni says I should write about that first time—and perhaps I will later, because why did I choose to get fat right on the most important date of my life?

I ripped the seams on that expensive dress. But then I was always outgrowing clothes—I grew so tall so fast!

Mother says I could open a secondhand store with the clothes I outgrow. Actually, I always save my thin clothes. It's the big sizes, the clothes I could never stand to have around, that could open a store.

Anyway, I digress.

This evening, watching the way Mother encourages Ben to eat and eat and eat, I see how I was a victim of her stupid, old-world ways. Mother, you fattened me in order to survive infancy and childhood and now you expect me to stay slim and attractive. Mother, I hate you for fattening me up and then expecting me to get skinny. I hate you for making fun of me as if you could embarrass the fat off me. I hate you for looking at me with contempt every time I reached for second helpings.

In blistering language, Harriet attacked her memory of her mother. Then, by sharing some of her bitterest memories with the Writercise group, and through the group's urging, Harriet continued to write through the anger.

Notes

Writercise 7:
Letting Go of Your Fat Past

This is not an exercise in hate, but one of letting out and examining that hateful feeling; then, rewriting—and replacing —the bitterness, bitterness that will turn to bile if left to sit in the gut too long. In Harriet's case, understanding eventually did displace much of her bitterness, as she could begin to see when she wrote:

> In my younger days my mother used to say, "Scrape your plate and the doctor can wait," convincing me that because I weighed twice what my classmates did, I was doubly healthy. I understand that she survived the sickly Depression but that was fifty years ago. It's a bit absurd at this point that she should think my son needs to be as big as a blimp to protect him from the invasion of foreign germs.
>
> I never really considered how the hunger of those Depression years affected her mothering. I guess I never realized how much I blame her for my big belly, and yet if I think of her when she was a little girl, young and afraid, eating bread with bacon drippings, sometimes day after day, I guess I can begin to accept that she did the best she could with me.
>
> Still, I can't quite forgive her, not while she continues to ignore my wishes with my son.

At another time, Harriet wrote:

Dear Mom,

You're to blame for the way I mother myself with food, only feeling complete when I am stuffed. You are to blame for programming me to bulldoze my way through food as if my health depended upon it. How can I switch gears now? I know you weren't all bad. You taught me how to sew and cook. I guess you never knew how to eat right either. You were just blessed with Grandpa's metabolism.

But Mom, I'm in no danger of starvation and neither is my son. I guess you can blame the Depression and your mother for the way you stocked me with surplus goodies. But Ben is not a wartime baby, so call off the reinforcements. I guess I am your postwar child. But Mom, I'm not a devastated country who now must be rehabilitated by a stern if loving overlord.

Harriet wrote until she was able to let her mother off the hook and take responsibility for her own future with food. First, however, she had to trace her anger back to its origin in order to let it go. Remember, when exploring old feelings, especially those of anger, the feelings must be written through completely in order to get beyond them to forgiveness and responsibility:

. . . You did what you thought was right. You wanted me healthy and, later, you wanted me happily attractive. You made mistakes, but you tried to do the

right thing. Now, if I want to be thin, I have to do the
right thing according to what I know about weight
loss. First, I have to quit blaming you and start relying
upon myself . . .

Thus Harriet was able to recognize her mother as the
formative influence. Yet, she also needed to divorce herself from
her mother's influence. Not that those feelings disappear forever. Instead, they become background for the choices you make
in the foreground of your life, for as Harriet continued:

Even today I feel like getting up and bowing
whenever I eat all my supper. And if that were all my
mother encouraged me to finish, perhaps I wouldn't
have to battle the bulge every day of my life. But now
at least I feel I have a real weapon . . .

Harriet's mother never did stop giving her son's clean
plate a standing ovation, nor did Harriet ever fully lose her
compulsion for fullness. However, Harriet claimed that the more
she traced blame back to her mother, the more control she gained
over her own food choices, as she came to accept her mother's
training as the unalterable past and her own present behavior as
the only part that could be changed.

Melissa is another, different kind of story altogether.
Melissa's big-city sister taught her to put two fingers down her
throat and vomit whenever she overate, years before most
people had even heard about bulimia. The big-city sis used the
technique very sparingly and thought she was teaching her kid
sister a survival tool for emergencies. However, Melissa decided

she'd found a convenient tool for weight control, sometimes employing it three times a week.

Through another, different kind of therapy group, Melissa had changed her bulimic pattern, but it was not until her diary work that she began to release her sister from blame, blame which went far beyond the bulimia. Melissa wrote:

> I blame Keri for being so perfect! How could I ever accept being the pudgy one with her as the pert and pretty kewpie doll from Mother's collection?
>
> In the beginning, every time I threw up I thought, "Soon I'll be just like Keri." Funny, but I think that eventually stuffing my face and staring at chunks of myself floating around in toilet bowl water released me from wanting to be Keri. Toward the end I would think of Keri doing this disgusting thing and she became a lot less perfect and a little more human . . .

From the back seat she'd long taken whenever her sister was present, Melissa wrote out her blame and found it led to putting herself in her own driver's seat.

Consider putting yourself back into your earliest memory of your family table. Remember who sat where and said what and then write through that memory.

Gisela's dinner table dilemma centered more around her father than her mother:

> I saw myself as the little kid at the dinner table. My father as usual glowering at me in disapproval. My

mother praising me for eating more than my skinny, pretty sister.

Both Mom and Barb would defend me from my father whom I always seemed to irritate unbearably. Perhaps he saw himself in me. Is that where those love-hate feelings stem from? Come to think of it, what little contact I had with my father was at the dinner table and this was almost all negative.

That was my family dinner table! Mother praising me for eating a lot and my father criticizing my bad table manners. No wonder I was forever spilling milk.

Interesting combination right there—shame and pride coming at me from both parents with me feeling guilt and pleasure.

Gisela says she knows she has a lot more work to do on her feelings about her now-deceased father. Writing out that ancient blame is a sure way to begin to carve a new future.

When you write out your own story of blame, in truth, it becomes your song of freedom, so remember to write in the chorus both understanding and love. Your mother (or father, sister, brother, or friend) is/was just another imperfect human being, playing his or her own off-key lessons. Write out your fault-finding dirges until you finally reach that unmistakable feeling that you've hit the right chord. You'll know it when you "hear" it—it's just the beginning of your own song of freedom.

Then write, write, write, until you "sing" the blame away.

Notes

Writercise 8:
Climbing the Family Tree

Let's start this one off with a little drawing lesson. Take a second to remember how you've drawn trees in the past. Tree drawing has got to be a universal experience. Whether with pencil and paper, brush and canvas, or a stick in the dirt, drawing trees represents our desire to re-create the life-giving growth of that most sacred and gifted plant on earth—the tree.

In drawing your tree, let yourself feel as innocent as a child with crayon in hand. Better yet, put this book down a moment and go look at a tree through the eyes of a child—your Skinny Kid or Chubby Child, if you will. Contemplate a tree outside your door or even outside the window of your car.

For a moment or a while, enjoy that tree. Sometimes just looking at a tree can feel like a real hike in the forest.

TREE 1: Your Family Tree

Draw a tree. Let it be a very special family tree of sorts. Trace each branch back to the trunk where other people, most often parents, have influenced the growth. Those influences can be represented as shoots and leaves, or even knots and bumps in the bark.

Write a description of your tree. Consider how you can make it better.

Every so often, as you write in your diary, take out this drawing of your family tree and add various fruits or blossoms to the branches. Let this new growth signify new behaviors that have improved your food intake and strengthened your eating patterns. Prune any branches that hinder growth. Allow the knots and holes in the bark to fill in naturally as the entire tree becomes healthier, more able to withstand stormy weather.

Consider this tree a visual aid for getting to the root of your eating disorders.

Along with this telltale tree, you'll want to write letters to the people who may have unwittingly twisted your branches —uh, shaped your eating habits.

Consider that root rot doesn't always lead back to another person. Someone may have started the tree's decay, but you haven't been spoon fed for a very long time, so beware of misplaced blame.

Take responsibility for your tree. Water it with at least eight glasses a day and fertilize it with natural foods.

TREE 2: Your Food Tree

Begin by drawing your food tree in your mind. First, close your eyes and imagine what your food tree looks like today. Is it twisted like a pretzel with too much salt? (Not to worry if it is, because all good fruit trees sometimes have twisted limbs.)

Is your tree tall, stately, and as full as an evergreen? Or short, slim, and graceful as a willow tree?

Imagine now the tree you want to be. A healthy, thriving, just-the-right-size tree.

When you open your eyes, begin to draw that tree, the one you want to be. Give it plenty of branches. On those branches, draw in the foods you know are the most healthy and slimming. Let yourself believe you have the power to design the diet to maintain that tree for the rest of your life.

Every mealtime call that tree briefly into mind before beginning to cook or eat.

Notes

Writercise 9:
Women Who Bake Too Much

There are probably as many reasons to bake a cake as there are to eat one. Women who bake too much are usually ones who eat too much, too. And yet, so often baking that cake is only the frosting on the . . . well, you get the point. Occasionally we might need to bake a cake, but more often, we just want to hang around the kitchen.

More than any other room of a house, the kitchen seems to belong to women. For many of us, it is our aromatic office, our creative cornucopia, our one and only cozy nook, the way to our own heart, our room of rooms, the place where others come to nourish themselves and worship us, the nook where the clock ticks backwards to our mother's time, and the part of the house our children will most recall as home, the place where we bake and bake and bake. We do it so darn well and that herbal essence of tea steeping or coffee brewing smells so good, so very, very good.

Again, you get the point.

When it comes to the kitchen, words can only hint at the power in our pantry. And the reasons we bake are as numerous as the analogies for the room itself.

How many of the following cake-baking excuses do you own?

- I'm baking this for the kids (husband, neighbor, women at the office).
- If I only eat one piece a day, it'll last a month.
- The mix was on sale.
- The recipe looked interesting.
- Since I made it, it would be a shame not to try an itty bitty taste.

- I can eat it now and work it off later.
- It's the smell, not the taste, I'm after.
- If I don't put nuts in it, the kids won't eat it.
- It's for company. There won't be any left over.

Can you add to the list?

In my own diary, as I weighed my cravings, I continually found other reasons besides the cake itself for the actual baking of it. I wanted to cook something rich and fluffy whenever I felt poor of spirit and one-dimensional in my writing. Whipping up some frosting was easier than whipping my thighs into shape. Sometimes I just plain needed to do something creative with my hands like rolling dough or weaving a lattice crust on the top of a pie.

When I started keeping my diary handy in the kitchen, I began to track my motives as well as outline possible alternatives. Gardening, for example, was something I personally enjoyed when I felt a need to be creative and handy. Admittedly, the great outdoors sometimes lacks the coziness of my wood-panelled kitchen and sometimes I feel as if I just have to surround myself with the smell and feel of dough rising and baking. Nevertheless, digging and planting in good, fertile dirt has replaced much of the routine baking I used to do.

Writercise students found some unique ways to circumnavigate their own choppy desires to bake. A lot of the cooking we do comes from our need to be creative and useful to others. But there are other ways to accomplish that.

One avid baker built a doll house for her daughter complete with miniature clay food stuff for the tiny cabinets and refrigerator.

Another woman who quit painting ten years ago, frustrated by the difficulty of selling her work, brought out her oils again. She now paints still-life renderings of those gloriously glossy illustrations in cookbooks and says if she never sells a single piece of art, the release she felt from the bondage to her oven is payment enough.

Still another diarist and gourmet cook realized that baking complex recipes made her feel smart and that she did, in fact, feel dull and uninteresting without her petite pastries and stuffed Danish delights. She enrolled in school to finish the degree in sociology she'd left hanging when she began a family.

By keeping a diary in a handy place in your kitchen, you can train yourself to bake a batch of alternatives in your allegorical oven. Every time a motive is revealed, say for instance you bake cookies for your children whenever you're feeling guilty about working too many hours, write out a list of possible activities that would show your children you care without sabotaging your own dietary needs. Also, unless you're including the children in the baking process itself, you're only taking more time away from them.

The best way to reveal your ulterior motives is to ask the right questions—repeatedly. In other words, ask yourself:

> Why do I want to bake at this moment?
> What do I get out of baking?
> Why do I want to bake this particular recipe?
> What appeals to me here?
> Who am I baking this for?
> If my diet could speak, would it object to this
>   recipe?
> Why do I still want to bake it?

When you know *why* you do what you do, it's a lot easier to plot other ways of getting the desired result. Outline some options in your diary and post them on your refrigerator and the next time you're ready to pull out the pastry cutter, scan your list for an option that would suit your present mood.

Liberate yourself from the consequences of cakes.

Notes

Writercise 10:
Thought for Food

You've heard people say that just thinking about food makes them fat or that all they have to do to gain weight is to look at food! It's probably because thinking about food is usually accompanied by eating it.

The truth is, thinking thin can keep you thin and thinking fat can make you fat, but not because the mind can actually pad the hips with imagined fat, although it seems to me that the mind does indeed have the capacity to convert mental images into solid physical realities. More to the point, however, thinking thin promotes the kind of behavior necessary for being thin.

People who fill their minds with food instead of thought should be doing just the opposite—filling up on thought for food.

What kind of thought can take the place of food? Lofty thoughts? Happy thoughts? Intricate or simple thoughts? Or perhaps reverent and respectful thoughts, probabilities and possibilities, philosophies and prophesies. Natural thoughts filled with the sound the wind makes as it breathes through the woods, bringing with it the trill of birds and the rhythmic flow of rivers?

The point is, you choose the thoughts you think just like you select the foods you eat. For some people, thin thoughts are full of logical conclusions like "ice cream pie × seconds + snacks = one humongous problem," while for others, thin thoughts can be as artistic as seeing oneself wearing a specific dress, dancing with lithe limbs to a particularly aerobic rhythm.

Thin thoughts. We all have them.

"I wish I were thinner!" is as common as buttered toast among women of substantial size. However, it is one of those thin thoughts that is imbued with frustration and self-recrimination. Replace it with "I am thin enough!" and leave your mind some space for dessert.

Like thoughts of a life lived thin.

Like thoughts of living life without thought of fat or thin, because thin choices are a process of natural selection. The Zen of thin means being one with thin, and I believe it is a birthright for each and every one of us, especially now with recent studies showing the correlation between greater longevity and thinness.

A healthy, balanced diet of thought is as simple as making a salad. You choose the ingredients, mix it up, and enjoy the fresh, crisp flavors in your mind. Substitute thought for food. Feed on ideas, considerations, and intentions. Bake up a flavorful fantasy and remember to select the thoughts that move you closer to your goal of good health, and thinness will occur naturally.

Eat imaginary food instead of the real thing.

When I suggested that my Writercise group feed on imagined food instead of real food, some worried that thoughts of food would only stimulate their appetite. Yet, in our society our appetite is continually stimulated by the media. Every check-out counter in America is surrounded by last-minute disasters of bite-sized chocolate and all-day suckers. Hardly a cash register stands without some little goodie waiting to ambush the best of intentions.

Think of Marlene with her mouth full of kitchen vernacular and her stomach ever ready to digest those tasty metaphors and spicy analogies. Even her diary was laced with aromatic terms:

I feel flakier than a pie crust . . .
I put my wants on the back burner until the kids were ripe enough to stand alone . . .

. . . His attitude was stiffer than beaten egg whites and his personality, twice as bland. Why did I feel it my duty to both soften and pepper him up?

. . . Even today I'm still trying to sweeten life for my kids. I'd roll them in confectioner's sugar if I thought it would help them out there . . .

Neurolinguistic programming claims that people relate to the world in visual, auditory, or cognitive ways. From the sounds of Marlene's diary, I began to wonder if there shouldn't be another classification for olfactory. Marlene seemed to communicate through smell and taste.

And the more Marlene dieted, the thicker she sprinkled spicy verbs and flavorful nouns into her journal. It was as if she was feeding her subconscious tastebuds with actual thoughts. Her mind was as hungry for the sensuous texture of food as her stomach was for the actual stuff. When this was pointed out during a Writercise sharing, Marlene began to make actual entries that allowed her to feast on literary food. Here's one of her examples:

Last night I wanted to eat the rest of the rice pudding in the refrigerator. I kept telling myself I wanted to fit into last summer's clothes more than eat pudding, and didn't touch it. Still I woke up thinking pudding. Maybe pretending to have had it will help. Okay, I ate the pudding. I lingered over each spoonful, closing my eyes and slowly letting the pudding dissolve, licking the back of the spoon. Oooh—I love the surprise splash of raisins, the lumpy texture of rice and eggs. I feel content and sweet!

And so Marlene nourished her hungry mind. For Marlene, pretending was enough. Since often it is the emotional comfort of food rather than any real physical hunger factor that stimulates desire for specific food, the imaginary treat can often suffice as a satisfying substitute.

At Marlene's urging, other starving minds began setting their own inner table with imaginary buffets. Most reported a cathartic effect and a diminished appetite. One woman compared it to a recurrent dream that often visited her whenever she dieted. A conveyer belt of endless food seemed to assure her that the foods she loved would not run out while she was filling up on cucumbers and watercress.

Like the subconscious solace of such dreams, writing can appease the sensual appetite in a peculiarly pleasing way. While Marlene found her cravings could not be ignored, they could be fed a steady diet of words that shaped quite nicely into hunger-appeasing images.

The next time you find yourself craving a specific food, try writing out a scenario where you indulge yourself in that food. (Save this one for times you are not physically hungry.)

Record your impressions, vividly and in detail—the way the food looks and smells, how each bite feels against your teeth, the tactile impressions in your mouth, the bursts of flavor upon your palate, even how each swallow feels, and the way the food rests in your belly—the cessation of hunger. Again, remember that scientists claim that the nervous system cannot differentiate between real experience and one imagined fully and in detail.

Most important, allow yourself to feel completely full and describe that satisfaction.

You may have to stretch your imagination on this one, but it is well worth the effort. You may find yourself forever cured of specific cravings, as Marlene found after she digested her own words:

I love the gritty texture of eggplant parmesan upon my teeth. The complex character of the food is like a great wine that improves and changes right in the glass. The pungent aroma fills the room even before I bring the fork to my mouth. And when I finally do, first I taste a tingle of tomato, then a cheesy, herbaceous zing sizzles my palate, until finally I get the subtle earthy flavors of the eggplant itself. I just love it! Which would be fine if I could eat a normal portion, but whenever I fry up eggplant I can't get my fill. Here in my diary, I can have my fill!

I gobble another piece too fast to really taste it, so with the next piece, I linger over the sauce and enjoy the way my teeth sink into the fleshy vegetable. The pungency of garlic spreads like wildfire inside my mouth and nose. I am content to nibble now. A nibble is as good as a bite. I can nibble a hundred tiny tastes and finally feel full. Fried eggplant parmesan remains my favorite dish. I can nibble to my heart's contentment. I still love eggplant parmesan, but I no longer feel like *I have to have it.*

Marlene claims to have found new meaning in the word "nibble."

Go ahead and try it for yourself. Nibble your own way through your favorite fatty foods to the thin, skim-milk center of your being!

Notes

Writercise 11:
Feasting on Joy!

Joy! Such a simple word. We can all define it. Dictionaries call it everything from intense happiness to mystical delight. A kill-joy is a low-down stick-in-the-mud who never jumps for joy and a joy stick is the modern equivalent of the all-American baseball bat. Joy! A candy bar was even named after it.

My favorite meditation, a "thinkercise" if you will, explores joy as if it were that part of the self which is super heroic. Superjoy is that part of me that "insists upon joy in spite of everything!"

While I was struggling with the lightweight theme of my first novel and healing from the heavy emotional weight of my knee replacement surgery, Tom Robbins, my literary hero of deep philosophical whimsy, wrote to me, saying "what we must do is insist on joy *in spite of everything.*"

Insist upon joy! In spite of everything! I loved it! I'd always wanted, sought joy, but had never been so absolute as to insist upon it. Joy leaves little room for self-pity or self-doubt; yet, I'd grown so accustomed to feeling both, that joy seemed as rare as Kryptonite. I needed an ultra ego, someone who vowed to fight for truth, justice, and the right to smile through scars. Someone who would fly flags, capes, and kites no matter the circumstance.

And so I invented Superjoy.

Superjoy breathes deeply enough to hold her head up high. Smiles come easier that way. Smiles and deep breaths help her stretch her spine tall, her limbs long and free of pain. Muscle tightens for super heroines. Although Superjoy was conceived in the intellect and born as a physical sensation, she quite miraculously developed into something very soulful. This creation of mine came as a kind of super comic relief to my once desperate character, finally rooting in my very being, as I sought to milk joy from the thorny, prickly, and downright painful parts of my life.

In other words, it was Superjoy to the rescue.

Superjoy is that part of all of us that seeks to taste, swallow, and digest the real joy in life—the pure beauty of a pristine valley, the wonder of clouds in the sky, the tiny insects in the grass, and the touch of humanity in our fragile fingertips.

By creating your own Superjoy you too can find the strength born of grace and prayer, happiness and hope, love and trust.

Best of all, you can rescue yourself from looking for joy in all the wrong places, particularly food.

Empower yourself with an inner vision of your Fat Lady and Thin Woman coming together to look for joy. You may call your Superjoy by another name, but her mission is to uncover real joy—not the kind you can stir-fry, buy, or win on "Wheel of Fortune." Genuine joy is generated in your mind, heart, and soul.

Write your own prescription for joy and then go fill it with the things you like to do, be, see, and feel. Yes, yes, I know that taste is as much a joy-producer as our other senses, but we who have used too much food to fill the spaces left by a lack of real joy have dulled our other senses and need to de-emphasize taste to balance out the scale.

When you meet and greet your Superjoy, you'll be guilt-free and can truly taste and enjoy healthy food. Or as Marla put it in one of our Writercise workshops:

Wow! I just had the world's greatest encounter with Superjoy, the heroine within. I saw and felt so much—I was really a lovely person with long, curly hair and a lavender leotard with a floating white gauzy cape. Toni's "menu of joys" was such fun to choose from. I ordered up a plateful of friendly conversation and a bowl of cheery romance for dessert.

It's so great to leave my negativity in the coat room and to realize I do have the capacity for self-fulfillment. My wishes really don't focus on my body. My primary desire isn't to be thin. It's to be serene. This workshop and my creating the time each day to really give to myself, especially taking the time for meditation, is reminding me that I have many spiritual strengths and powers.

I am enjoying learning more about how my mind creates my reality. I don't need to step on the scale, for it only slows my progress to find I have not lost as much as I think. Feeling slim and good about myself is far more important than how much I weigh. Funny thing is, whenever I feel thin, people ask me if I've lost weight.

Marla liked my Superjoy meditation so much that she made her own meditation. She imagined herself as a child going to the store, buying a *Wonder Woman* comic book, and then becoming Wonder Woman. She imagined going to a power lunch with Gloria Steinem, Betty Friedan, and other strong-minded, powerful women whom Marla admired. The women at Marla's imaginary power lunch affirmed her good work—what she had done in her life and how powerful and beautiful she really was.

For weeks afterwards Marla reported that she questioned her cravings for fat-filled foods by asking herself, "Would Wonder Woman eat *this?*"

So go ahead and let yourself create the super heroine within you. Though I choose to call her Superjoy, you may call her anything that embodies inner power and high-spirited joy-fulness. Close your eyes and imagine yourself as a super heroine.

Dress Superjoy any way you wish. Let her don some-thing spectacular. Superjoy goes to lunch in the most wonderful restaurant imaginable. A waitress brings her an appetizer menu. The list of entrees ranges from a hot bubble bath to a stroll through a fragrant meadow. Let yourself study the menu. You'll recognize each item as one of the genuine, simple pleasures in life. Don't read any further. Stop and picture the entrees in your mind. Close your eyes for a short time.

Now open your eyes, pick up a pen, and describe what you look and feel like as Superjoy. Next, draw a word picture of the place you chose to partake of your Superjoy's scenario. Now, describe your "Simple Things in Life" menu.

Writercise diarists have shared all kinds of down-to-earth appetizers like running, swimming, hiking . . ."hiding out in the tall grass with a crossword puzzle," "brushing my hair a thousand strokes," "skipping work to sleep the afternoon away," "watching the rain from a second-floor veranda," and more.

There seems to be no limit to easily accessible joy. And that's only the appetizer. Go ahead and eat from a steady diet of simple joys, one bite at a time, for the rest of your life.

Now, getting back to Superjoy at that most wonderful of imaginable restaurants. Let yourself visualize a waitress bring-ing you another menu, a menu of main courses. The items here are a bit more elaborate with side dishes and condiments. The choices are also a bit more nebulous, if equally delicious. This menu encompasses the larger picture, including who you are, and who you want to be, and what you want to do with your time and energy. The things on this menu might seem more like peace than joy—or success—or any number of the possible positive pursuits life offers.

So go ahead, again close your eyes a moment, now and often throughout the next few days, weeks, or even years. Ask yourself, "What is the main item on my menu?"

Don't forget to make your choice more real and concrete by putting it down on paper—and then pursuing it with all you've got.

Finally, we come to my favorite part of Superjoy's feast. Now we get to order dessert! Don't you feel a lot like a kid when you think about dessert? I do.

Dessert. What is dessert?

Dessert can be all the sweet, doughy, crusty, crunchy, nutty, fruity-tootie, good 'n gooey stuff forbidden to us, not because we're not kids, but, "Well, frankly, adults just don't do things like that," or could it be you think you don't deserve dessert?

If so, let it go. Think about dessert in a whole new light, beyond the glare of the reflection in the fridge. Think of dessert as the sweet, delicious center in the adult who once was a child and loved singing "Row, row, row your boat" in three-part harmony.

Ah, dessert! Hard to say it without smiling. Umm-umm, dessert. Before you read any further you might want to put down this book, pick up your own diary, and describe which of life's bounties you might consider as part of the frosting on your cake.

Now that you've played with some words yourself and written out a few dessert suggestions, consider what other Writercise diarists found on their dessert menu:

> petting cats and dogs,
> giggling like a little girl,
> walking under waterfalls,
> watching a fire warm me and my husband inside a
>   cabin somewhere in the north woods,
> reading the grandchildren a bedtime story,

dancing in candlelight,
watching the moon rise over the mountains and the
   sun set over the ocean,
river rafting,
skinny dipping,
sail boating in a nice safe bay,
playing piano once again,
finding a dry piles of leaves waiting to skydive into.

The dessert selections are as numerous and unique as kernels of caramel-coated popcorn.

And, remember, you won't get any dessert if you don't write it in on your own menu and then order it up in front of you!

By the way, that last dessert item, written as it is, seems more like a still-life portrait of possible joy. If Amanda were to order this entree and follow it to the letter, she would find herself watching the waiting leaves!

Amanda's dry piles of leaves waiting for her to skydive into are just that—dry, waiting leaves. The neurolinguistic mind is quite literal. But perhaps Amanda wrote it that way for a reason—she was afraid of skydiving. Amanda later rewrote that spicy, if dangerous, dessert into something she wasn't afraid to sink her teeth into. She saw herself "tumble into scattering leaves on a bright fall day." Now, whether or not Amanda actually skydives before tumbling is another story that only Amanda can decide.

Let yourself tumble into the truth of your own personal joy! Your own super heroine will take to the sky!

Notes

7

Making Love

Our Beaus, Our Bodies, and Our Self-images

Why do we give men (or for that matter, each other) the power to judge our beauty contests? I'm not just referring to those glittering extravaganzas and county fair events, from "Little Miss Diapers" on up to the "Queen of the Universe."

It's the day-to-day judgments and comparisons that do more harm to the average woman. From the time we first noticed the cute smiles underneath the crew cuts of those people who were kind of like us, but also kind of different, we've vied for their attention, seen ourselves through their eyes, and cared what they thought about how we looked.

Oh sure, in the limelight of our liberation, we know that looks aren't everything, or for that matter, even half of everything. If we accept ourselves as a trinity of body, mind, and spirit, then our bodies might logically be a third of who we are, but certainly not the sum total.

Basically, we liberated ladies like to think of our bodies as mere shells for the more important stuff, like inner spirit, intellect, and the expression of both.

Even so, the majority of us have been—or still are —affected by the opinions of our male counterparts. We sometimes dress for their smiles, diet and sweat for their approving gazes, and feel as fat or as thin as they imagine us to be.

And yet, rather than playing a game of blame-and-rage, we need to be examining our own place on the board. After all, destiny is more than a roll of the dice and a lot less fated. Once we learn to play by and even to bend the rules, we can make our moves more in tuned with what we wish to win and are willing to lose.

Notes

Notes

Writercise 12:
Soothing the Ego-Ache

Begin to explore your male-female issues in your diary. You might be both surprised and relieved at what you find.

Consider Annie's situation. Twenty-six-year-old Annie felt inferior around her husband. She blamed him for her lack of confidence, for he was often critical and, as Annie put it, "always ready for me to screw something up." Annie was certain that he had caused her feelings of inferiority. Annie also feared Charlie would realize his mistake and divorce her.

As Annie began writing about those feelings, remembering a time in her early marriage when she hadn't seemed so clumsy and unsure and he wasn't so ready to criticize her fall, Annie wrote:

> The more he carped and quibbled about my driving, cooking, or for that matter my ability to stay with a diet, the more inadequate I felt. But it also seems that the more I fumbled, the more critical he became and then, the more insecure I felt.
>
> During our college days, he admired the way I could whip term papers out at the last minute or balance plates up my arms at the Hungry I Cafe. But I always felt like I was duping Charlie. The real me was far clumsier and less accomplished. The real me was that C- student at Southside High.
>
> I was so graceful back then, my boyfriend's sister gave me dance lessons for weeks before giving up and telling me to waltz a lot.

In truth, I wasn't very surprised when Charlie began criticizing me. I guess I expected it. Maybe even thought I deserved it. Why?

At my suggestion, Annie began tracing those same feelings of inferiority inspired by Charlie, or perhaps played out around Charlie, back through some of her high school sweethearts. When she wrote about the few boys she dated and the fewer ones she "went steady with," that same gnawing self-doubt riddled her writing:

> . . . I never really felt like Anthony *liked me* the way he liked Liz for her pretty face or Susan for her smarts.

> . . . Other boys were in love with their girlfriends, but they showed it in ways Lenny never did around me.

Annie tracked her feelings backwards until she remembered her first crush, and subsequent ego-ache. It was her cousin Robert who started her primping before the male mirror.

Annie expressed a fondness for Robert. However, between the lines there is an undertone of hostility over his "strutting, selfish lifestyle."

As she wrote about the "tacky women and stupid girls" he'd bring to family gatherings, her tone got younger and younger with each remembered episode.

I suggested Annie pursue this younger voice. Annie stretched even farther back into her memory by writercising the alphabet with her left hand. ("Wrong-handed" writing works well in stimulating memories of younger times because of the connection to that earlier struggle for controlled penmanship.)

Annie grasped her pen as tightly as Little Annie might have—and this is what Big Annie uncovered:

> Me and Bobby are with my other cusin. [*sic*] She picks her nose, ugh. We are eating at his mom's little table with some other cusins. Bobby is in between me and her. He puts olives on his fingers and lets her bite one off. Then he goes and gets mad when I take one from his dish. He wouldn't dare eat an olive from her nose-picking finger. I hate them both. He likes her better. I want to cry. Instead I call him stupid and eat olives off my own fingers . . .

This was her first peer-oriented ego-ache, and there were other similar episodes, not necessarily with Bobby, but other little boys and later younger and older men. Also, these negative feelings were reinforced by a critical father (Annie is still writing about this, her primal ego-ache); otherwise Little Annie might have written a different story. As it was, Annie's relationships continued to re-create that early ego-ache, each time trying to make it better.

For most of her life, Annie allowed one little boy's fickle feelings to interfere with her love line. Now, with the help of her own diary insights, Annie felt self-awareness feeding her sense of self-worth.

"I feel better just seeing how silly it all was and is and how easy it is to believe I deserved that olive off his plate—and I've been mad at him ever since."

Although the group suggested Big Annie call her grown "cusin" and tell him just that, Annie declared that knowing is enough.

Annie was right.

The point of sifting through early ego-aches is not to wallow in the sandbox. Writercising can be an effective exorcism if you allow yourself to pick up each memory and hold it to the light—turning it slowly, studying all sides, and finally letting it drop back into the sand.

Why do such seemingly small ego-aches affect some of us more deeply than others? Diary writing doesn't necessarily unravel the entire mystery, but it certainly shines a spotlight on the hidden drama of day to day reality, providing clues, avenues of escape, and sometimes just a few minutes behind a locked door where the kids can't burst in, demanding you fix this or find that.

Writercising about our beaus, our bodies, our self-images often requires an understanding of the past. Try tracking your romantic history backwards and letting go each and every heartache along the way. Of course, if you can instantly yo-yo back to those young, young days, by all means, scribble away.

For now, take some time to begin writing about your present relationships with men. So much of our opinion of ourselves as women, especially as sexual women, is tied up in the experiences we have had or continue to have with men, and even earlier, with boys.

Sure, in many ways the males of the species are just like us. They eat and sleep. They speak our language and they walk upright on two feet. They laugh and if they're lucky, they even cry. And yet, in many other ways, men and women are worlds apart.

In my novel-in-progress *Shoes of the Mermaid*, my young heroine Mimi laments the difference by crying out,

"Sometimes I wish I were a fish with no legs and no—you know what!"

Men sometimes act as if they left their emotions at the bottom of the sea. But, as an older, wiser Mimi learns, "to live in the fullest tide of ebb and flow, fulfillment and benevolence, we women must learn to reach the empathetic tide between the sexes. And to touch the line that separates us is to grasp and hold, examine and understand the things that join us as well."

The common points of our experience as cultural beings, as human beings, all await us somewhere on our common horizon. But, then why's it so darn tough to share it with men?

Yes, Mimi, men and women are different. Why do you think they are called the opposite sex? Yet, as many a diarist comes to understand, they are just like us.

Gisela, the Writerciser who was teased for being taller than the boys in her neighborhood, concluded:

> My ex-husband always seemed so perfect, so
> cocksure! All through our marriage, I worshipped
> him. I gave him the power to walk all over me. In my
> eyes, he could do no wrong. Now I know he's a
> fallible human just like me. I've been angry for so
> long at boys and later men. Clint made his mistakes
> but so did I. I went from husband worship to hating
> men with very little in between.

Gisela is now learning to accept herself, her hopes and fears, artistic dreams and human frailties, and in so being, perhaps will meet a man who can respect and love her for who she is. And yet, if that never happens, she will not back down from her feminist pursuit of her own humanity.

For Gisela it was easy, if painful, to track her female-to-male history to a point of self-acceptance. For others, such crystallized perception comes only through much soul-searching.

Write to that man (those men) in your own past. Write long willowy, loving letters, as well as short, sharp hate-mail.

Write a Dear John letter or two.

Play with the idea of men as mirrors and see what you come up with.

Write out the details of your latest fight with your current boyfriend, mate, or husband, while it is still fresh in your mind and you are still smarting from the sting.

More than trying to remember who said what, try to feel the experience again. What feelings about yourself did that disagreement stir in you?

Trace those feelings back to another boyfriend where similar feelings arose. Write about those feelings until you've exhausted the subject. Pose the question in your diary, "Who was I involved with before this man, and why does he stir similar feelings?" Wait quietly. (Sometimes days or weeks will pass before a face or a name comes to mind, and eventually another pulse will be felt, and then you can trace your own heart backwards through your romantic history.)

Write in the voice of your Chubby Child and Skinny Kid. Yes, both. If you have made contact with your Fat Lady and Skinny Kid, then surely you can comprehend these other two characters beneath your surface.

Of course, never feel pressured to be as analytical as Annie wrote above, or other Writercisers. You may need only dig as far as last year to resolve the tracks of your own tears and reroute yourself to a more loving destination. Those early ego-aches were only stops along the way to your true self.

For rare it is that the Love Train is a nonstop express rolling past constantly beautiful views. Often there's no palatial cabin or even a comfortable berth for our lovemaking, but there is a free ticket in your diary and a map to anyplace in your heart.

Remember, love and/or marriage is not a one-way excursion into Happy Ever After.

Notes

Notes

Writercise 13:
Stuffing Your Feelings, Stuffing Your Stomach

Marla, the perceptive writer who, in an earlier chapter, traced some of her food-obsession roots back to mother-inspired insecurities, also began to analyze her marriage within the balanced light of her diary. Two years into a second marriage which she considered quite successful, Marla found herself stuck in an alarming, if incomprehensible trend she was able to deny no longer—she'd gained nearly a pound for every month she'd been married!

Marla's increasing girth seemed to have no effect on the love and devotion of her new husband. It was, however, a problem with Marla who told me she felt her self-esteem shrinking as her size was increasing.

Unlike her issues with her mother, at first Marla didn't see much connection between her weight gain and her relationship with her new husband.

"He tells me at least once a day that I'm beautiful and that he loves me. He's never once criticized me for gaining weight," Marla told me. Then she laughingly added, "Of course, he does get irritated when I don't get his socks matched right or there are spots on the silverware."

Marla dated Brad for three years before their marriage and she knew he was a perfectionist who sometimes yelled his frustration when his world let him down. Yet, Marla was amazingly tolerant of his outbursts. His good qualities far outweighed his one character flaw, she rationalized, and as a middle-aged divorcée with a half-grown and sometimes still difficult family, Marla felt she was no prize herself.

"Whenever there's a real problem, Brad is the best friend I've ever had. He's a wonderful listener, he gives good advice and ever since our first date, he's been willing to get involved.

"So how important is it that it that he yells at me once in a while when he's had a bad day and I've done something stupid like let his clothes mildew in the dryer?"

Like most of us, Marla made mistakes from time to time. She didn't need Brad to verbally "beat her up" for them. Marla was good at doing that to herself because she knew how it worked. Her verbally abusive mother and her loving father who made excuses for her mother's behavior had shown her how.

But Marla's mother had never apologized for hurting her. Brad was different. He hated his outbursts as much as Marla did, and he always apologized for making her feel bad. One of the reasons he loved her so, he told her, was that she was such a good sport. Marla didn't try to hide her hurt or her concern, but she didn't rub it in either. And although she'd been keeping a journal and writing about her weight issues for years, she didn't see any psychological connections between the weight gain and her marriage.

Yet, excerpts from Marla's own "Fat Lady Diary" indicated otherwise.

Dear Fat Lady,

Brad and I hit it off right away on the phone. The dating service gave us a chance to have a meeting of the minds before our bodies ever came into the picture. It was a shock to finally meet and find that Brad was only an inch taller and probably just a few pounds heavier than myself—especially because I'd just starved myself into a size 8. For weeks as we developed our wonderful friendship, I felt awkward standing beside him because in my head I was still a size 16. Brad never made weight an issue, but one of the first times we made love, he said something about what a great body I had—"although I know you'd probably like to lose 20 pounds."

It was hard to tell him that I'd just *lost* 20 pounds and the real Marla was a size 16. I guess one sign we were on our way to a real relationship was that I did tell him. I have to admit I was relieved that as I slowly regained the 20 pounds during our three-year courtship, he remained loving and supportive.

Did I gain the weight back deliberately? I don't think I did, but maybe I was testing his sincerity because I know I kept thinking, "This will end when he sees the real Marla." We did break up for a few months, but it was a matter of "commitment anxiety" on his part he said, rather than any dissatisfaction over my appearance. Still, I wondered.

When, after a few weeks of separation, he instigated a reconciliation of our relationship, there were never any more questions about commitment or concern about appearance. We still rarely talk about my weight and it's always been very difficult for me to share with him just how ugly it makes me feel.

About the time Marla began to face these issues, Brad and she had the worst fight of their young marriage—a fight she says they both now recognize as a turning point in Marla's sliding self-esteem. Marla shared the details in the next Writercise class.

Marla and Brad were excited about making all-new Christmas decorations themselves and were working on it together, only she couldn't decide how to sew some lace on the bells so she went to Brad for advice.

"I thought you knew how to sew," he said, much too loudly. Frustrated, she tried to explain why the project wasn't working as easily as she'd planned, but instead of listening and helping, she felt Brad treated her as if she were stupid.

Suddenly Marla was screaming, "I hate you! Leave me alone! F—k off!"

The outburst was completely out of character for Marla. For just an instant Marla thought he might hit her—or maybe it was Marla who would attack. Then they both retreated, Marla to her sewing machine, sobbing and wondering why. Although she'd never said anything like that to her husband before, the whole thing felt so strangely familiar.

Later in her journal she wrote:

> He doesn't understand how, just like Mother, he
> makes me feel so awful. In some ways this all started
> with the Karen Carpenter story on TV. I'd watched it
> alone and been very affected. He couldn't understand
> why I was crying over a "woman sick enough to
> starve herself to death." I tried to explain my own
> feelings about eating disorders and having a fragile
> sense of self-worth. We usually talk about everything
> so easily, but I felt shaky talking about this. It seemed
> important to share "feeding" issues with him, but
> somehow very risky. He said it was the first time I
> had told him I have low self-esteem—I can hardly
> believe that.
>
> Then a few hours later, the fight. It feels like I
> revealed how shaky I am and then instead of helping,
> he went for the jugular, making me feel stupid over a
> silly sewing project. It's not the first time that my
> admitting a frailty has made him angry. (What is it in
> him that can't handle my weak self?)

And Brad's anger feels too much like
Mother's. And Mother always made up for her
outbursts by baking a special treat for me.

Marla says that her husband and she were able to talk over their fight, both admitting they had problems with self-esteem and anger. To Marla, Brad's anger felt "like a little monster nibbling away at our happy marriage," while Marla's anger seemed more like a cry baby that needed to be "subdued with frequent feedings."

She explained, in the tenderest of tones, how his temper stemmed from the abuse he endured as a short boy and how "yelling is his way of protecting himself." (I always find it curious that many of us will extend to our beloved more compassionate understanding than we accord ourselves and our own pasts.)

Marla felt that tracing her love line back through earlier relationships improved her present marriage.

She still continued exploring her issues, claiming that the insights gained by writing in her diary have helped her to "turn off" her desire for desserts, as well as look at food more like bodily fuel than emotional pabulum.

Marla was kind enough to send me an update of her writercising self. (Thanks, Marla.) After the workshop, Marla continued writing in her journal, trying to work out some new life goals for herself. She continued dealing with her childhood issues (at one point seeking professional therapy to help her sort through her feelings).

She began to risk being more open in her confrontations with Brad, and for a time the marriage was under the siege of stress. Brad went to two therapy sessions with Marla, and together they have a much better understanding of how their marriage system works for them.

Brad still gets angry, Marla still gets depressed, but they've learned not to let a little emotional dip turn into a full-fledged crisis. According to Marla, both of them are slowly becoming more responsible for their own emotions, and the occasional flashes of mutual anger no longer threaten their marriage.

As she says, "A fight is no longer scary because now it's just anger, not hurts from thirty or forty years ago or even fears about future fights.

"I've learned to express my own anger without escalating, and he's learned that sometimes he can just walk away from a confrontation. We both feel more grown up."

Marla also reports that once she stopped repressing her anger at her husband and her own lack of productive work, she broke her pound-a-month weight-gain pattern and began losing weight.

One year after attending the Writercise workshop, Marla wrote to tell me that having completed her second semester of college "re-entry" course work, she's ready to tackle graduate school—and a sensible weight-loss diet plan.

She recently joined "Slim for Life," a group sponsored by the American Heart Association, and is slowly but surely losing weight. Marla also reported that writing to her Fat Lady and Thin Woman continues to inspire and motivate her.

Notes

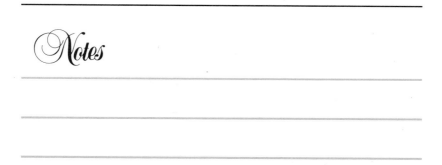

Notes

Writercise 14:
Big Daddy and the Original Ego-Ache

Of course, any woman who traces her boy-girl tracks back far enough will eventually stumble upon that primal ego-ache.

Yes, that original ego-ache is Daddy!

Yes, Daddy-ego-ache, because even if you were lucky enough to be born of a kind and loving father, you still couldn't have him all to yourself. He loved Mommy differently than he loved you. To a Daddy-adoring little girl, that difference may easily be interpreted as *better.*

And that is where all good boy-girl diary work should lead.

Back to Daddy.

Begin by writing letters to Daddy and see where those letters lead. Or, like one group of musical writercisers, write a song to Daddy.

Our father-root is as deep as the one with our mothers, yet we rarely dig beyond the topsoil of our father-daughter relationships. There are many cultural and emotional barriers to exploring, expressing, and thus releasing feelings about "Daddy," and so most of us live our lives making minimal contact with our fathers.

Although this is the nature of a paternal society, nature is always open to a little shift, even in her granite mountains.

Writing letters, mailed as well as unsent, can give you a chance to explore the rockiest of long-forgotten ledges of your father feelings, deeply submerged like the ocean floor.

During a recent Father's Day weekend, one of my Writercise classes decided to write some poetry and songs to Daddy. Lyricism is a wonderful way to approach the lesser-known, possibly more threatening situations because poetry, "therapoetry," allows us to hint at emotions, use symbols, be as sketchy as we need to be.

A great many diaries have been shared with me by the women in the workshops, and I've read enough to believe that a diarist will never unveil more feelings than she is capable of handling at any given time. I've also come to believe that therapoetry allows a greater freedom than any other written medium for exploring fear—and of course for expressing joy.

The following pieces come from many diverse diaries. (My most deeply felt gratitude to my writercising muses for allowing me to share these here.)

Cookie Jar Thief

Daddy, quit hiding cookies
please! The quilt gets ridiculous
and so does the way you tease me
for my big butt and hippo hips.
Please Daddy, quit hiding your
heart! The longing makes me hungry
for the love in the cookies you hid
when I was just a skinny little kid.

This was written by a woman whose father had recently died:

daddy o' daddy, you taught me dignity and how to die
a little bit every day because daddy o' daddy i
watched you die and daddy o' daddy, i've been
watching you fade from my arms ever since that first
day you held me in yours because daddy o' daddy, the
older i got the less you held me, until the end, daddy,

when i barely opened my arms to you and daddy o'
daddy how i wish we could try again and i'd snuggle
under your warm smile and smile into your sad eyes
and never ever grow up

oh, daddy o' daddy, I guess I'd do it all again,
grow up
grow old
and watch you grow away
to somewhere I cannot yet follow

And this one came from a woman who was trying to let
go of feelings that she disappointed her daddy:

Dear Old Dad

Good ol' dear ol' Dad
I remember the shine in my patent leather shoes
and the one I sparked in your eyes when I was
a bright and obedient little girl

Good ol' dear ol' Dad
my Mary Janes got dusty from dirt-biking and
    dancing
and I'm no longer the apple of your eye
but tough old fruit leather in your side

Daddy Boy, New Daddy O
look beneath the patent leather to the little
    girl inside
I'm still your spark of love
gone off to ignite hearts and hearths of fire

Therapoetry can be the song your Thin Lady's been waiting to sing, whether the lyrics express longing, loneliness, disappointment, or pain. And if the emotion you feel is anger and you need to rage, there's no friendlier medium than meter and verse. It's the nature of poetry to lead you either through rhyme or free verse to freedom from your burdensome feelings, and more often than not, to forgiveness and joy.

Although many of us deal with a father who is not there for us emotionally, Eileen's father was absent from the beginning. Although there was a stepfather later on, when Eileen was eleven, the daddy-desertion blues had already set in. Eileen simply expected men to desert her. At thirty-one, she certainly had a heart-breaking history—three marriages and all but one ex-husband being somewhere between Timbuktu and God-Knows-Where, despite the three children they left Eileen to raise alone.

Eileen, a big, beautiful woman, admitted that she probably got big to save herself from getting involved in another losing marriage. Whenever a man paid attention to her, she headed straight for the refrigerator. Like all of us, Eileen wanted a loving daddy; however, her history, riddled as it is with big ego-aches, keeps her ambiguous—and overweight.

When Eileen started a Writercise workshop, a sales representative she saw every few weeks had been pursuing her with lunch proposals. Recently he'd stopped asking and Eileen had started wondering whether she really wanted to live the rest of her life alone inside a refrigerator. So, she began to write:

> If only I could be sure he wouldn't love me and leave me. I know it's foolish and impossible, but I want a guarantee from the one thing in life that can't even keep a promise.

Eileen had a lot of unexpressed feelings toward her original deserter, the father she'd never known, and I suggested she begin by writing letters to him. Eileen filled up half a notebook with her little girl rage. Although Eileen wished to keep most of her diary private, she did share the following entry:

> All my life I missed my father. I missed him at graduations and birthdays. I missed him thirty-one times on Christmas morning and for thousands of bedtimes. Mother was great but I always felt only half-kissed and half-tucked in.
>
> I missed him and I know it!
>
> I wonder about him, though, because I don't think he knows to miss me. And I suddenly feel that there is a lot about me worth missing . . .

Eileen's circumstance may be an extreme example of desertion. However, desertion often happens even when a parent lives under the same roof. With busy careers, many little girls never see their fathers outside of mealtimes. They often bring feelings of desertion to the dinner table.

Old family dinner dynamics can linger long after the table is cleared. Forty-three-year-old Jean wrote:

> I think I learned to stuff my feelings like Dad did. Mom would complain about me and he would eat. Dad wasn't going to save me from my mother's anger. He disappointed me. He could have stood up to her . . .

Marla reached into her father connection through her domineering mother.

> Mom, I don't know what you were so unhappy about
> —probably because Dad was so chauvinistic—kind,
> but still a chauvinist who never allowed you to be part
> of any decision. He never let you grow up and I guess
> you were in a rage at him all my life. I didn't
> understand why you nagged him so, why meals were
> so often ordeals. I know I sided with him and wanted
> to sit after dinner talking with him instead of helping
> you in the kitchen . . .

Marla said that she was always reluctant to get up from the table. Maybe Marla still longs to hang around the dinner table and talk with her dad. I suggested that Marla go ahead and have those conversations in her dairy. Even though Marla's father is now deceased, there is a catharsis in letting your pen alter your feelings about the past, filling in the silences with words that should have been said a long time ago.

Notes

Notes

Writercise 15:
Guess Who's Coming to Dinner?

Let yourself wander back to your early childhood dinner table. Re-create a mental image of those mealtimes. Let yourself remember who sat next to and across from you. See your mother and father in their regular positions around the table.

Listen to your own heart. Try to hear the words you would have spoken to your father had you the insight then that you have now. Write those words to him.

Now listen hard for the words your father could have replied. The words you so wanted to hear. Write them down as if those words were really spoken.

At another time, let yourself relax and remember that early family dinner table. Be a silent observer and watch the interactions between your mother and father. When they converse cordially or argue angrily, how do you feel? What do you do?

Kelly felt like she could change the direction of her parents' fights by drawing their attention away from their bitter words and toward her. Kelly became the family klutz:

> I knocked over my milk so many times I finally had to drink it at the end of the meal and then only when my mother stood over me and watched me drink it. For years I wasn't allowed to keep a drink in front of my plate . . . Even today, when someone raises their voice at dinner I'll drip sauce or something else on the table.

It's as if by staining the tablecloth with bright food colors, I spill out my own inner turmoil. On the one hand, I'm stuffing my emotions down with food; on the other I'm spilling my guts all over the tablecloth, but since I'm too ladylike to actually spill my guts, I spill whatever else happens to be handy.

Notes

Notes

Writercise 16:
Mirror, Mirror in Your Mind

Let yourself be the fairest in the land.

There is no magic formula for reflecting thinness in the eyes of one's beloved. But there is one genuine way to be beautiful—and that is to feel your own, unique beauty, inside and out.

So often we look to the mirror to confirm some preconceived image of ourself. Words like fat and ugly stare back at us because we expect it from our mirrors. Sometimes we make impossible comparisons to the faces and figures in magazines.

To release the hold such modern-day icons have upon our self-esteem, I recommend tearing out a picture of a fashion model and writing to that picture, for example: "Yes, I'm jealous. Yes, I wish I could look like that in a bathing suit. Yet, why do I believe you're also smarter and nicer than me?" etc. And remember, picture-perfect women probably represent less than one percent of the population. Be kinder to your own image. Every time you look in your mirror, find some compliment to extend to your image, even if it's just that you have the same nice eyes or shiny hair you've always had.

For quite often, our mirrors speak harsh words. Perhaps that's because we listen for the slander.

Someone else, perhaps a love interest, may have slanted our perception of ourself. Perhaps your diary might reveal your mate has a prejudicial preference for a model-thin body, which is an unnatural expectation for you. If so, your choices are not limited to starving yourself to suit the model mold or leaving him and finding someone else. Try to open discussion with him, and ask for a little understanding. And remember that empathetic line—men are as much victims of modern-day model worship as we women are.

Start redefining your image by paying attention to the things men say about women. Movies and television are a great place to start. Write down the things that rub you wrong, whether it be adulation of a beautiful woman or snide comments about Fat Ladies.

In the movie *Body Heat,* the William Hurt character makes reference to Kathleen Turner's beauty no less than twenty times. Or consider the ridiculous message in the *Nerd* movies. Even the leading nerd hero somehow winds up with the luscious leading lady!

Listen for comments made by strangers in the street and men in the workplace.

Listen and write. Record your feelings. Write them out until you feel free of their twisted hold upon your heart. You may just find yourself discovering and discarding the meaningless, useless, hurtful misconceptions you had adopted without even knowing you were believing in them. Here are just a few examples:

> . . . I never realized how my favorite soap opera star had me believing that beautiful is better.

> . . . My husband jokes all the time about really obese women we see. I used to laugh even if I was crying on the inside.

> . . . Why aren't there any plain or chubby teen-agers in situation comedies? I'd rather watch "Roseanne."

Write away all the full-of-bologna, beauty-and-the-beast, "she's a real dog" myths you've ever bought and paid for with your self-image.

Then, the next time some jerk jokes about fat fannies, or some movie star melts at the sight of a lovely looking lady, you'll be able to keep from recording a misguided message and playing it back in your mirror.

When you look in your mirror, look into your own eyes and ask yourself if there are any negative comments made by the men in your past which linger and cloud your vision of yourself.

Any little ego-aches?

Any butt-ends of jokes that aren't funny anymore?

Any big slurs?

Little lies?

Slanted mirrors?

And speaking of slanted mirrors, in my Fat Lady Blues poem, I jest about my mother slanting her mirrors backwards to thin down our images so that we can eat more of her marvelous meatballs. In truth, I slanted my own mirrors backwards.

I wanted to have my cake and eat it. Yet I wanted that thin image as well.

By the way, I still occasionally take my full-length mirror and slant it flatteringly backwards, especially when I start feeling fat. Those taller, thinner angles comfort and encourage me to keep eating healthy, balanced meals and to keep on dancing.

And since I believe we project on the outside what we believe we are on the inside, a little planned self-deception can sometimes be as healthy and healing as words on paper.

Go ahead. Redefine your mirror image. Talk to your reflection. You've heard about the benefits of taking the time to talk to plants, how an encouraging tone helps them thrive. So, why not take a moment to say something sweet and encouraging to your own reflection?

Let yourself play with mirrors.

Visit a house of mirrors and laugh at the delusions inherent in pieces of glass.

Play dress-up and watch the little girl inside ham it up.

Pretty soon, you will begin to enjoy not just the words you write, but also the sight of your own self.

Give yourself permission to apply a little self-relish to your sandwich. Lord knows, there's been plenty of horseradish slopped on over the years.

Remember, you deserve to like your outer reflection as much as your inner resonance.

Mirror, mirror in your mind, are you fair to yourself? Are you kind?

Though the answer lies within you, look to your mirror for a clue.

Notes

Notes

Notes

8

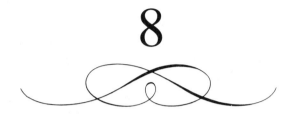

Making It Fun

Hunger: The Unwelcome Guest

Hunger. What exactly is hunger? Undoubtedly, it's a physical sensation, a built-in warning that starvation is possible and a gnawing reminder that food is a daily necessity. In many parts of the world, sadly enough, hunger is a constant companion, even a death sentence.

For women who diet, hunger is but an uninvited, unwelcome guest. For us, hunger is a growling, thoughtless child that tugs and clings to our apron strings while we resist baking chocolate chip cookies.

Hunger wears many disguises from boredom to loneliness, to fear and stress. Writercisers have defined it as an emptiness, a gnawing, a nagging, a rude visitor, a restless rumble, a self-doubting about as useful as the center of a doughnut.

Hunger is often the Bad Boy of the stomach, the Runaround Sue of the menstrual season, and the Midnight Messenger for refrigerated leftovers.

Whatever metaphor we wrap around hunger, it can make or break the dream for healthful thinness.

When I suggested to an early Writercise class that they befriend their hunger by writing letters to it, I never expected Hunger to answer back. Ah, but that's the energetic freedom in the river of words! Words, once started flowing, often meander into channels where they can restock a staggering pool or even bring a dried-up valley back to life.

Helen set out to befriend her hunger by asking for an explanation. "Why am I so hungry?" she asked, for although she usually ate a balanced lunch and breakfast and even a fruit snack before leaving work—a 7 a.m. to 3 p.m. shift—Helen was plagued by a desire to devour fatty starch during the few hours before her husband arrived home.

Often not waiting until she reached home, Helen hit the bakery or one of the fast-food restaurants on the way home. Or if she made it safely past the little convenience store and into her driveway, then she often gorged on leftovers or even "boring bread and butter." Sometimes she munched on whatever she was preparing for the evening meal. Often she wasn't even hungry at mealtime, but she always sat down and ate again with her husband—"just to keep him company."

Since Helen didn't want to plan an after-work activity, her Writercise cohorts suggested she prepare supper the night before so that she wouldn't be in the kitchen during those tough two hours. Helen also rerouted the ride home to eliminate all but the convenience store. To get past that, she was instructed to talk into a tape recorder, beginning the writing session that was to continue until hunger subsided.

Helen thus began her conversations with hunger:

I'm aware of you there in my stomach. Lay off. Leave me alone. I want to forget about food until Jeff comes home. Can't I feed you the idea of me, happy in my shorts? Can't you see how all this fatty food hurts my heart! I cannot cure you with food. [Helen was a nurse.] Too much food will only keep me tired and worn out when Jim comes home. Can't you wait until suppertime?

After writing this particular passage, Helen said she went outside to read and relax. However, Hunger would not be filed away in those few, short sentences. Even though she'd just eaten an apple, Hunger grumbled for more. And so Helen picked up her diary, intending to write it away when Hunger took an active voice.

Quit blaming me for getting you fat. It's not fair. You're always mistaking me for discontent. That emptiness at the bottom of your heart isn't me. There is a lack in your life but it is not necessarily a lack of food. Look to the rest of your life before you start filling in the blanks with food.

Helen shared that entry in a Writercise class, although she resisted exploring the more debilitating lack in her life—the emptiness of something beyond her stomach. Expecting instant results, Helen became disappointed when her diary hadn't yielded a quick and easy solution and she went back to afternoon munching. Six weeks later she was still a victim of her hunger, as motivated by food as ever.

I saw Helen a year later. She'd gone back to writing in her diary and was, she said, writing daily to her hunger. I don't know whether or not she'd dropped any weight, but she certainly seemed much lighter of spirit.

Instead of trying to silence her growling hunger, she'd begun listening to its cues and writing down specific plans of action.

Helen said her hunger was motivated by a lack in her marriage. Now that her children were grown and out of the house, she needed to refigure their marriage.

By addressing her hunger as if it were a tangible part of herself, Helen wrote into the core of it. Yes, it took her some time to address the real issue—her marriage. However, once she did, the voice of her deeper hunger came to her assistance.

Perhaps this is a good time to encourage anyone who does uncover something too powerful or painful to handle alone, even with the assistance of a friendly diary, to seek appropriate help. Professional therapy and responsible, established weight-loss and/or eating disorder groups, such as TOPS (Take Off Pounds Sensibly) or Overeaters Anonymous, the later being a free, support group based on the Twelve Steps of Alcoholics Anonymous, can help you through the darker moments of self-discovery.

Another way to use this book is to form your own Writercising group. (In the back of this book, I've included a copy of a contract for your use as a device to help keep your group on target. Feel free to copy it or rewrite it.)

Notes

Writercise 17:
Hungry Helpers

Begin to reprogram your thinking about hunger by writing to it. Ask hunger to define itself. What else besides a physical desire for food motivates your hunger? Wait for a response and try dialoguing back and forth with your hunger. Listen to it. Understand it. Release yourself from the slavery of serving it continuously with food.

If you are eating a balanced, low-fat diet, the length and depth of the hunger you are likely to experience is a far cry from the haunting hunger of the physically impoverished. Those with a social conscience may wish to donate the money saved by eliminating snacks to organizations that help people who cannot befriend hunger because it is their constant companion.

Letting yourself feel and question and finally befriend hunger can free you from a lifetime of fighting it. Simple hunger can become a comfortable physical emptiness, a condition of temporary want which allows you to truly savor the nutritious meals you do eat.

Moreover, treating hunger like an experiment, something to be studied and understood, allows you to differentiate physical from emotional hunger. And that knowledge is a powerful tool.

Describe hunger as if it were a living, breathing character outside of yourself. Give it a name. Write a letter to your hunger. Ask it to explain itself on the pages of your diary.

Reread the pages in chapter 2 on the Nitty-Gritty diet plan or design your own balanced diet. Write out a schedule and stay with it despite your hunger. Every time you do experience hunger, write to it. Ask it questions. Wait for responses.

Hunger can become a friend, if you welcome it as a concrete sign that your body is burning calories and fat.

Redefine hunger. Thank your hunger for assisting you with your plan for thinness. Always remind yourself of its temporary nature, keeping panic at bay. Remember, as long as you are following a healthy, balanced food plan, you cannot possibly starve to death.

Write a poem to your hunger.

Have fun and write a silly ditty to your hunger. I wrote the following light verse when I first learned the difference between my emotional and physical hunger.

> who's this grouch in my belly
> crying for garlic vermicelli
> forever yelling to be chock-full
> of nuts and doubts and crammed-dull
> meal after meal, an endless conveyor belt
> rolling me away from thin and svelte
>
> who's this sad-sack in my soul
> begging bread in her alms bowl
> as if I weren't an overfed worrier
> a caviar dreamer and hungry courier
> hoping for a fat-free and fun farm
> sowing thin thoughts that transform

Despite the intimidation that classic literature often bequeaths the practical thinker, poetry building can be an exquisite experience, turning ideas into a fun, freeform mix of art and therapy.

For now, forget the Emily Dickinsons and the Walt Whitmans, the e. e. cummingses, and other learned poetic voices who may have stilled your own metric verses. Sign and stamp your own poetic license with your official seal as head diary writer.

An excellent primer for any would-be poet is Shel Silverstein's books, *Where the Sidewalk Ends* or *A Light in the Attic*. Although found in the children's section of the book store, browse through them for their simple structure and for the funky fun of it. No other modern poet, to my knowledge, better demonstrates how the most common of subjects sometimes makes the most insightful of poetry.

Remember—

Hungry Hanna once thought it hip
to fill me so I could not zip
my fears loose nor pants tight—
not if I took another bite . . .
ah! but Hungry Hanna saw the light
one word is worth a thousand bites

The reason poetry is so therapeutic is that while you are searching for the right word to fully express the feeling in your gut, you are contemplating that exact feeling and focusing on understanding just exactly what it is that has moved you to write it down.

So go ahead, write a haiku to your hunger. Glut yourself with rhymes and meter, words that succinctly speak to that empty feeling in the pit of your stomach. Or simply write free verse with no preplanned structure in mind at all.

Write your own Ballad of the Hungry I Cafe.

Notes

Writercise 18:
Lost and Found in Space

Save this writercise for a star-filled evening. First go outside and look at the stars. Quit thinking and just look. As soon as you finish reading this sentence, close your eyes and imagine yourself one of those stars—a bright light, aglow with being part of the big, beautiful night sky.

Great. Now try to let that feeling stay with you for the rest of the night and into the following day. Write about it in your diary; think about it when you're driving to work.

Save the rest of this writercise for a few days later when the sky is blue, even a patch of blue will do. Now look up at the same sky that was once filled with stars and find a cloud to contemplate. Get your mind into that same star-gazing mode, but this time imagine yourself a cloud drifting lazily through the sky, nary a worry nor a thing to do except be a cloud. So, when the time comes, close your eyes and feel yourself being that cloud. Be that cloud.

Now again spend the next few days drifting in and out of being a cloud. Remember, it takes only a second to be a cloud.

(I know it seems silly, but imagination is your inner child's best friend and the pure child loves to pretend and look at clouds.) So go ahead, write about the feeling—be as cumulus or nimbus as you wish, remembering that what you write in your diary belongs only to you.

No one else ever has to know that you were once a cloud or a star. Have fun with it. Don't worry what the point of it is, although there is, in fact, a point—simply enjoy exploring the expansiveness of space.

Where does all this spaciness fit into writing yourself thin?

If you can expand your inner space, it may be easier to reduce your outer space.

Continue romping through that inner playground of images and ideas. Allow yourself to imagine being slightly crowded into an elevator with other people of various sizes. Picture all the other people as somewhat thinner than you. Again when this sentence ends, close your eyes, and feel the others around you; feel your own body and the space it occupies in that elevator and the impressions your body makes being part of this crowd.

Well done!

Now imagine the elevator stopping and letting on another person—a person somewhat larger than yourself. Ride that elevator up another floor in your imagination by closing your eyes when this sentence ends and focusing your attention upon that new person sharing the elevator with you and asking yourself what you feel—whether you experience resentment, anger or indifference.

Then imagine the elevator stopping at yet another floor. Everyone but you and the larger person stays on. The two of you ride up another floor. Again closing your eyes at the sight, explore your feelings—are they any different now that the others have gotten off the elevator?

While the feeling is still imprinted in your body, write about that elevator ride. How did you view your own body? Can you note any specific feelings about the space you occupied?

Describe any of the other people who stood out in your mind. How did you feel about the larger person? The thinner one? Any marked differences?

After conducting a similar meditation in a Writercise workshop, some interesting impressions and reactions were recorded. Feelings of discomfort, even guilt, were not uncommon:

. . . I tried to squeeze myself smaller, so I wouldn't crowd the others.

. . . My body feels too big to be in here. I feel panicky and want to press the button to leave.

. . . Maybe if I hadn't eaten pancakes for breakfast I wouldn't have to suck in my stomach.

A common hostility was also evident toward the largest elevator rider. Sometimes it was expressed as an "embarrassment for" this new person getting on the elevator. Although we discussed the possibility that even a thin person coming onto an already crowded elevator would provoke some resentment, it did seem that size triggered a more intense reaction:

. . . One of her takes up three of them. She should have waited for another elevator.

. . . I think of the really big people I see in the street and recall overpopulation and how small the world is. Why can't she diet? Why can't I diet?

. . . I hope she doesn't stand next to me . . . I don't want to see myself in her.

. . . I want to grant her the same rights as the others, but if I feel ashamed to be fat in this thin world, then surely she should be twice as embarrassed.

Now take a moment to consider a cloudy sky, a starry night, and a crowded elevator. As far as the space you occupy, do you have any less or more rights than a cloud or a star or a very, very fat person on an elevator?

Try to keep this up front in your mind whenever you feel oppressed by size or space.

Finally, practice expanding your sphere of influence by drawing concentric circles in your diary. As each circle widens to encompass more and more space, tell yourself you can occupy as much or as little space as you wish. Whatever actual space your body fills, you deserve it.

Drawing concentric circles can also be a simple yet powerful warm-up for writercising. Although circles within circles seem, at first, to represent something wound and tight like a spring or a screw, your control over those circles allows you to unwind any inner tension. As you draw, direct yourself to let go of guilt and other negative emotions. Allow the hypnotic circular motion to sooth and relax, remembering that the number-one cause of overeating is tension and the more tension-relieving activities you give yourself, the less tempting surplus food will become.

This writercise is as accessible as doodling.

Draw circles around your tension and rings around a rosier disposition.

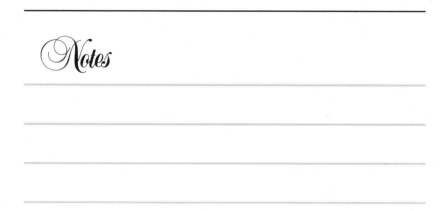

Notes

Notes

Writercise 19:
The Bigger I Get, The Better I Feel

Pat was the director of a halfway house for delinquent boys. She was also active in civic affairs, on numerous boards, and a popular speaker for various fund-raising and social events.

In other words, Pat was a leader—a leader who claimed to have learned early on that it wasn't always easy to command attention in the body of a thin (i.e., frail) woman. She went to an all-girl high school where her natural affinity to be in charge was unaffected by her sex.

Yet, in the coed world of college and work, Pat's authority was challenged again and again by men and even other women who were taught to put their confidence in men competing for the top banana's spot in the fruit bowl.

And so Pat said, she became larger and larger in order to be taken more seriously:

> . . . And so I cut my long, superfluous hair and shortened my name from a playful Patty to a no-nonsense Pat. I also got fat. I think I believed that I was able to project power in my weightiness. Although I never admitted it to myself, I believed a big woman should be taken more seriously than a lightweight one. More than anything, I want to be taken seriously. Fat is serious. Thin seems like so much fluff.

It is not uncommon for women who struggle in an uneven system to try to balance the scale by adding more weight to their side.

Before you absolve yourself of such prejudice, consider the feelings a thin woman in a position of authority evokes in you. Would you feel safer in a dangerous situation with a big, burly policewoman or a thin pretty one? Does this value judgment necessarily follow through for their male counterparts?

Begin to contemplate and write about your own prejudices. Choose a favorite activity, something you are skilled and capable enough to imagine teaching to others.

Now imagine your Thin Woman instructing a group of others in this favorite activity of yours. Include both men and women in this fantasy, making some of them younger and some older than yourself. Next, consider whether your Fat Lady would feel any more or less able to lead this group. Do you expect to be equally received and respected?

What about imagining a different kind of activity, one that is not traditionally expected of a woman? What kinds of feelings do you expect to encounter from other women? From men? What in your Fat Lady makes this new role easier or more difficult?

Write down your impressions. Since a lot of our own judgmental feelings lie hidden even from ourselves, write often upon this subject.

Pat found some release from the subjugation of her Thin Woman by writing scenarios where she performed her leadership duties in a thin body.

I'm speaking to the Board of Realtors about growth containment. I'm pretty thin. I'm even wearing my hair long again. I'm panicky because the man in the chair across from me is staring at my thin body and smiling like we're on a date. I feel pressed to make him smile instead of just giving him the facts. I'm nervous like it is my body that is making this presentation and my mind has nothing to do with the value of my words.

Now I breath deeply and tell myself it's okay. My thin body isn't here to impress anyone but myself. I know my material. Men and women who refuse to take me seriously have their own hatchets to bury. But not in me. I'm as powerful now as I was in my fatter body.

Remember, writercising is very much a freeform dance. Now that you know a few basic steps and can write in a Fat Lady or Thin Woman voice, stretch your imagination by playing both roles at the same time. That is, write a dialogue.

This bigger-better writercise is a good one for dialoguing because gaining or losing personal power usually engenders an inner dichotomy. It's easy to imagine that it is always one part of us that wins and another that loses and thus easy to imagine a conversation between a powerful self and a weakened wisp of a self.

Your power play may not read like Pat's. You may even feel a complete reversal of types. Perhaps your Thin Self has more confidence and therefore more power than your Fat Self.

Consider Denise's "Thin is better" dialogue:

DENISE BIG:	If only I could lose weight. I'd go back to school and get my master's.
DENISE THINNER:	Why can't you get it now?
DENISE BIG:	I don't like to get up in front of people looking like this. Graduate school means a lot of presentations.
DENISE THINNER:	I'm scared of talking in front of groups too.

DENISE BIG:	Yeah, but people trust what thin people people say.
DENISE THINNER:	Which people? You?
DENISE BIG:	Maybe I do. Maybe I trust thin more than fat.
DENISE THINNER:	I'm thin and I'm you and you're me.
DENISE BIG:	That's right. But most of the world trusts thin more than fat.
DENISE THINNER:	Then let's prove the majority wrong. Let's enroll in school while you still own our body. Be as powerful as you can. I will help you. I will loan you my confidence and you can loan me your hunger.
DENISE BIG:	Sounds like a good working arrangement.

I don't know if Denise ever went back to school. Hopefully, she knows she deserves to get what she wants.

Go ahead, talk among yourself on the safe playful pages of your diary and discover another passage through the dark, perhaps a new vein into the pulse of your own personal power.

Notes

Notes

Writercise 20:
Classic Poetry in Motion

Roseanne says she loves to dance but that her husband never takes her dancing. She hasn't danced in five years—not even in her kitchen!

No doubt dancing with a partner on a real dance floor with live music, mirrors and strobe lights brings out the Ginger Rogers in all of us.

However, if Roseanne loves to dance, then she should dance.

If you love to dance, dance alone if necessary. (It's actually quite liberating.)

Dance while stirring the family stew or mopping the floor. Grab one of your children's hands and bop them off to bed. Dance circles around the dog and square-dance the cat into a corner. Dance under the bright lights of K-mart (out in public you may want to waltz rather than watusi, but then again, in the mad rush for polyester and plastic, who'd notice one lone cha cha cha?)

Or if you love to dance, slither into nothing but a naked fantasy in front of your favorite video and sway away. Stomp with frustrated outrage while the news drones on. Better yet, turn the music on and the lights off and dance in the dark. Light a candle for Little Egypt and shimmy in the solitary glow of your own footfalls. Twist the yoke from your twinkle-toes and lindy little bits of your life away.

Because if you don't take the music by the horns and bolero away your blues, you've no one to blame but your own two feet.

Sure, it would be wonderful if your husband pinned a white lily on your red dress and twirled you around the local hot spot. It also would be wonderful to win the lottery, yet that doesn't stop you from going to work every day.

And if you love music, you'll never really dance alone. Musical appreciation invites you to hold hands with Harmony and rest your head on Melody's notes. Close your eyes and feel rhythm flow in pleasurable waves through your body. And then just move. Music is your best dance teacher. Let it take you through the steps. And while you dance, feel like a thin woman or a proud thin bird. Stretch into the music and tighten up as the old Archie Bell and the Drells song "Tighten Up" exhorts.

Remember, all you have to do to climb on board the soul train, the dance express, is climb into comfortable clothes and express yourself. Two steps forward or one step back!

For there are as many reasons to dance as there are craters on the moon. Speak your moods through the gesticular language of pulse and sway. Listen to your inner music. Perhaps you need a little rain dance to tap your well of tears, or a high-stepping war prance to stomp on a few fears.

Whatever your mood, put some music on your stereo. Listen to the deeper rhythms, feel the persuasive sway of a saxophone or the contemplative thump of a conga drum.

If you love to dance, then delight in the vibrato of man-made sound. Moreover, be open to the natural possibilities of music inherent in nature. The ebb and flow of water, the song of birds. Or listen carefully to the first wind instrument, the breath of nature wandering over the planet. Long before our ancestors carved that first flute, the wind was blowing music through the reeds of swamps and hollows in the forests.

The natural music of the world is a meditation in itself. At your earliest inspired convenience, do a little experiment. For an entire day, pay attention to the sounds around you. Is there anything in your world that can be heard as a kind of music? You have to really listen and relax to catch some of the more subtle nuances of natural music, yet sometimes if you really relax and listen, even the rush of traffic can take on the tone of a wind instrument.

Listen to the way boot heels clap down a corridor like a timbale drumbeat. Keep a diary handy all day and take note of anything vaguely resembling music.

What has the natural rhythm of the word got to do with your pursuit of thinness?

Isn't it stress and anxiety that causes most of your overeating? Most modern women complain that their busy schedules limit the time they can spend diary writing or even dancing a mop around the house.

And so seeking musical harmony in all experiences can relax you, thus reducing your appetite. Seeking your inner harmonic voice can synthesize a hectic environment into something that is not only easier on the ears but the heart and soul as well. Even the improvisational jazz of the street can stimulate a relaxed mood. Think of the quintessential jazzman on the street. Cool, calm, and relaxed.

Begin by feeling the tiniest rumbling of joy. Feel it begin in your stomach. That's right—imagine your stomach rumbling, yet this time with joy instead of hunger. Don't panic if you cannot feel even a pitter-patter of joy. Relax and wait. Joy is often as subtle as a lettuce leaf.

Who knows what you could accomplish in the search for inner Joy. Everything from creative fulfillment of artistic dreams to the luxury of love are within Joy's reach, Joy's realm.

So now, right now—quit reading and thinking and begin listening and moving.

As Chissie Heins advised, "Dance like a Russian ballet! Dance like a twentieth century [fe]male."

Notes

Writercise 21:
Deep-Down Diary

How does one develop personal power?

I think of personal power as the ability to re-create the self—body and soul—in the image and likeness you most respect and admire. Since a body can only stretch and shape to a set range of physical possibilities, it's important to understand and accept the actual capacities and limitations of your body. (In view of some of those physical limitations, isn't it nice to think of the soul as infinite?)

The soul of course is always the toughest subject to broach in writing, or for that matter in any physical form, because after all, if the soul were physical, we wouldn't have to separate it into "body and soul." However, a deep-down diary makes an attempt to bridge the territory between the two. That is, an inner journal attempts to reach the realm of the soul through a visualized diary.

This is not to say that the act of physical writing does not tread upon soulful ground. Often, writing does filter the soul through the fingertips. However, even with long-winded, truly inspired writing, the hand eventually tires of holding the pen or the fingers lose their train of thought as they glide over the typewriter keys.

Yet, when you tire while writing in what I call your deep-down diary, you may simply fall asleep. Sometimes you may even finish the story somewhere in the symbolic library of your dreams.

What then is deep-down diary writing?

In my mind it is a form of prayer. Although I believe the best prayer is wordless, pictureless, and completely still, most often that nirvanic state eludes me and I must settle for a very human method of inner communication, like words or pictures.

Because I learned to pray the Catholic school way, I tend to think of prayer as a silent visual poem. In my youth, I silently mumbled the memorized words someone else wrote. Later, when I learned to let myself feel and think and express, I substituted my own words for rote recitation. My best prayers are illustrated. That is, I picture the state of being I wish to create as already existing in my mind.

Although I often think in pictures, I still prefer to pray in words. I created my deep-down diary by closing my eyes and telling my body to relax. I breathe in an even, circular pattern which helps relax me more. Next, I imagine myself walking down a long hall and opening a door to my inner writing room.

I created this room to suit my personality and you should do the same. Whether you are the big pillows and white carpet type, or the hardwood floor and rolltop desk kind of fantasizer, take a few moments to create the room you would feel most comfortable visiting. Remember in your imagination, an expensive leather sofa and priceless paintings on the wall are as free as dreams.

Sometime, soon after this inner writercise, write down a description of this room in your real notebook. The act of physically reaffirming what you create in your imagination strengthens that picture in your mind.

Once you have your inner writing room set in images, invite a diary to appear. Wait, confidently knowing you do possess an inner journal. Again, design the diary of your dreams and get a clear picture of it in your mind's eye. What does that inner diary look like? Remember later to write a description in your real journal.

For now, back to your internal diary, watch your hand turn the cover and open to a blank page. Watch yourself write, letter by letter, some special motto or affirmation for the day.

Writing in my inner journal has become a morning ritual. I usually jot down a line or two—something to guide my day. I try not to prejudice my lines, that is, only when I open my book do I seek the written words I need.

At my best, I allow the lines to bounce up from my subconscious spring of self-knowledge. After all, inner journaling is an open-minded endeavor. The meditative state of inner writing keeps my analytical, critical mind from laying its own trip upon my pen.

Needed themes will begin to occur and recur, expressed in simple, childlike form. These themes often redress certain self-doubts.

> I like me.
> I am good enough! (I am thin enough!)
> I deserve to be happy.
> I can succeed.
> Other people like me.
> I love me just the way I am.

I realize that many times, the opposite of these positive statements were written many years ago in the notebook of my youthful self-image. I began scanning my diary, looking for those anti-themes. When I found one, I'd imagine myself ripping out that page, tearing it into pieces, and tossing it into the garbage. As you get more familiar with your own inner journal, you too will discover some negative notes to yourself. You may not remember writing, "I do not deserve to be happy" or "I never succeed." Nevertheless, during more downbeat moments, you were very busy recording a sorry song of yourself.

Absolutely nothing appears in your inner journal that you haven't put there yourself. Most often those words were originally spoken to you by someone else—a parent, teacher, sibling, or some other influential person. However, you accepted them as truth and traced them into your soulful notebook.

You can see why opening your inner journal during the highly self-aware state of meditative silence can redress old stories while stimulating your imagination to write new ones.

Let yourself wipe your slate clean of "I can't," and fill it with as many "I can's" as you may need.

As a matter of fact, one of the simplest and most powerful beginning "innercises" you can do is to open your inner diary every morning before even opening your eyes and write "I can, I can . . ."

Because you can.

Be aware that the inner journal is much more subtle than words can describe. Except for a few intensely visual people, most innercisers find that words do not jump out at them. Rather, as they imagine their own hand turning page after page in their diary, they get a sense of something disconcerting.

If this happens to you, stop turning pages and continue breathing in a circular rhythm—and wait. Soon the words that describe the negative impression will be seen, heard, or felt in your mind.

Once you have thrown away that imaginary piece of paper, always remember to write the positive statement that counterbalances the self-recrimination. Don't be an empty revolutionary who overthrows the present government, yet has nothing better to establish in its place.

These days, I am a much more disciplined inner than outer diarist. Nonetheless, I continue to need, and use, the concrete dimension of exploration and revision that my paper notebook offers.

Also, since the inner journal is always the last of many meditations in the Writercise workshops, I have only limited feedback upon its universal utility.

However, one woman, who has remained a dear friend ever since her participation in the workshop, says she too wakes to her inner journal and that it calms her. A much more prolific innerciser than I, she makes inner lists of goals for the day and claims that often some forgotten item on her list will pop into her mind at the most unlikely of times, but that she forgets appointments a lot less frequently these days.

So, as you continue writercising, try adding some relaxed inner journaling to your program of thinking thin.

Write a glowing statement about fruits and vegetables or an inspiring word about walking.

Jot down a quick, aerobic phrase about jumping for joy, and a raving review of the new body you've created for yourself.

And remember, "Happiness—To get the real and lasting kind, you have to grow it in your mind."

That's far more than a great definition for thinness or living a simple, happy life.

It's a creed of freedom!

Notes

Notes

Notes

Epilogue

Dear Diary Readers,

My editor suggested I write you this letter, a sort of personal summation and "so long" song. I must admit the idea put me into a slight panic.

Why?

Ah, well, as I begin to write, I begin to understand why I feel threatened by a last heartfelt letter to you.

I feel a need to tie up the loose themes of this book into a neat, fancy bow, as if this outpouring and inputting truly has been a gift I wish to give other women who suffer from the Fat Lady Blues.

Yes, I am proud and excited to be wrapping this up for you.

Yet, like the Little Drummer Boy, I am afraid my gift is not good enough. And in this turn of phrase, I come to know that anything drummed from the heart is good enough. This book, dear readers, is full of my very heartbeat—a human heart with all its imperfections as well as lovely rhythms.

In writing to you, I come to understand that all along, I was fooling myself. I am not giving you this book. You, my Imagined Reader, gave it to me.

For even as I wrote that first entry to my Fat Lady, I sensed your understanding. I believe that what I have wrapped up inside this gift is the burden of my shame.

For when it comes to food, I have felt as guilty as Eve biting into that forbidden apple. I have carried so much shame. Shame over chocolate treats and cookies, cookies, cookies. A foolish, undeserved shame indeed, but a powerful shame all the same. A shame that will certainly take an entire lifetime to completely reshape into the loaf of the forgiving bread the Holy Man once multiplied and divided for all humanity to share.

Dear Diary Reader, thank you for your gift to me. Writing my own story, my own "Diary of a Fat Lady," has indeed healed much, if not most, of my own hunger and hurt.

Ever yours,

Toni Lynn

Toni Lynn Allawatt
May 1991

WRITE YOURSELF THIN

Commitment of Participant

- I understand that this is a six-week workshop and agree to attend each session, health and weather permitting.
- Since the premise of this course is learning to feel and think thin, I will not express my weight goals, either verbally or written, in terms of pounds while I am in a group session. (I am, of course, free to write about weights and measurements in my journal.)
- Each session will require some writing. This is my solo safari into myself. I will try to express my real feelings without regard for other people's opinions.
- After each written exercise, I may wish to share what I have written. I am free to decline reading aloud and will respect another's right to decline the same.
- No comments will be permitted during the times when another group member is sharing her/his diary. Afterwards those who wish to respond to the reading may do so, given certain guidelines to be established by the group. For example, only "I" statements are allowed. ("I" statements do not include "I feel that you . . .")
- Advice and criticism of another's feelings achieve nothing. I agree not to judge another diarist's writings and/or feelings. (Statements such as "You are too . . ." or "You should or shouldn't . . ." are examples of such judgmental statements.)
- What is shared here with the group is strictly confidential. I will respect other participants and their feelings.

Participant's Signature_____Date_____

Notes

Notes

Other Books for Weight-Losers from CompCare Publishers

Compulsive Overeater, *The Basic Text for Compulsive Overeaters, Bill B.* An interpretation of the Twelve Step Program for overeater by a nationally known speaker. Also includes chapters on abstinence, anger, fear and depression, relationships, money, switching compulsions. 00091, hard cover, 288 pp.

Maintenance, *The Twelve Step Way to Ongoing Recovery, Bill B.* This companion to Compulsive Overeater helps readers learn to live well, feel good, and maintain weight loss. Highlighted by personal stories of dramatic change and maintained recovery. 00208, hard cover, 352 pp.

Laugh It Off, *The New "Humor Strategy" of Weight Loss, Jane Thomas Noland.* Foreword by Dale L. Anderson, M.D. New theories relating appetite suppression to endorphins, brain-generated chemicals, give new meaning to this classic. If laughter and positive thoughts can raise endorphins, this fun-to-read book – with its clever, sound strategies and cartoons by Mimi Noland – will have readers laughing all the way to their goal weights. 04283, paperback, 300 pp.

The Thin Book, *365 Daily Aids for Fat-free, Guilt-free, Binge-free Living, Jeane Eddy Westin.* This weight-losers' classic, with 150,000 copies in print, offers a year's worth of empowering messages that strike at the heart of the problem – sagging motivation. 03046, paperback, 372 pp.

The Thin Book 2, *Winning Strategies for All Weight-Losers, Jeane Eddy Westin.* A collection of more daily messages about taking charge of your life, weight, and health through key principles of right eating, exercise, and positive attitudes. 03210, paperback, 384 pp.

Thin Is a State of Mind, *Nancy Bryan, Ph.D.* "Your body is a visible expression of the state of your entire being," Dr. Bryan says. She shows how to tap the power of your "thin mind-set," to begin to remove personal obstacles, relieve stress, and live more serenely – and coincidentally become thin. 03269, paperback, 192 pp.

Order Form

Order No.	Qty.	Title	Author	Unit Cost	Total
04383		Write Yourself Thin	Allawatt, T.	$11.95	
04283		Laugh It Off	Noland, J.	$ 9.95	
00091		Compulsive Overeater	Bill B.	$16.95	
00208		Maintenance	Bill B.	$16.95	
03046		The Thin Book	Westin, J.	$10.95	
03210		The Thin Book 2	Westin, J.	$10.95	
03269		Thin Is a State of Mind	Bryan, N.	$ 9.95	

Subtotal	
Shipping and Handling (see below)	
Add your state's sales tax	
TOTAL	

CompCare® Publishers
A Comprehensive Care company

Allow up to 4 weeks for delivery. Send check or money order payable to CompCare Publishers. No cash or C.O.D.'s please. Quantity discounts available. Prices subject to change without notice.

SHIPPING/HANDLING CHARGES

Amount of Order	Shipping Charges
$0-$10.00	$2.00
$10.01-$25.00	$3.00
$25.01-$50.00	$3.50
$50.01-$75.00	$5.00

Send book(s) to:

Name _____

Address _____

City _____ State _____ Zip _____

☐ Check enclosed for $_____, payable to CompCare Publishers

☐ Charge to my credit card   ☐ Visa ☐ MasterCard ☐ Discover

Account # _____ Exp. date _____

Signature_____Daytime Phone _____

CompCare® Publishers
A Comprehensive Care company

2415 Annapolis Lane, Plymouth, MN 55441
To order by phone call toll free (800) 328-3330.
In Minnesota (612) 559-4800